your guide to
arthritis

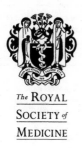

The ROYAL
SOCIETY of
MEDICINE

your guide to
arthritis

Dr Michael Snaith
MD, FRCP

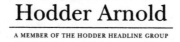

A MEMBER OF THE HODDER HEADLINE GROUP

Hodder Arnold have agreed to pay 50 pence per product on all sales made of this title to the retailer at a discount of up to and including 60 per cent from the UK Recommended Retail Price to The Arthritis Research Campaign.

Orders: Please contact Bookpoint Ltd, 130 Milton Park, Abingdon, Oxon OX14 4SB. Telephone: (44) 01235 827720, Fax: (44) 01235 400454. Lines are open from 9.00 to 18.00, Monday to Saturday, with a 24-hour message answering service. You can also order through our website www.hoddereducation.com

British Library Cataloguing in Publication Data
A catalogue record for this title is available from the British Library.

ISBN-10: 0 340 926015
ISBN-13: 9 780340 926017

First published   2007
Impression number   10 9 8 7 6 5 4 3 2 1
Year   2010   2009   2008   2007

Typeset by Servis Filmsetting Limited, Longsight, Manchester. Printed in Great Britain for Hodder Arnold, a division of Hodder Headline, 338 Euston Road, London NW1 3BH, by Cox & Wyman Ltd, Reading, Berkshire.

Hodder Headline's policy is to use papers that are natural, renewable and recyclable products and made from wood grown in sustainable forests. The logging and manufacturing processes are expected to conform to the environmental regulations of the country of origin.

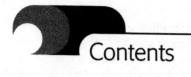

Contents

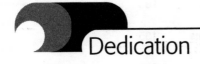

Dedication

To Penny
For her love and patience

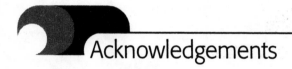

Acknowledgements

My thanks to Judy and Chris Williams,
Mike Cowley, Helen Coster and Janice Bryan
for their generous help in reading and making
suggestions to the manuscript.

Acknowledgement

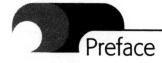

Preface

This new book, published in partnership with the Royal Society of Medicine, provides detailed, useful and up-to-date information on arthritis. It contains expert yet user-friendly advice, with such practical features as:

Key Terms: demystifying the jargon
Questions and Answers: answering the burning questions
Myths and Facts: debunking the misconceptions
My Experience: how it feels to live with, or care for someone with, this condition.

Bearing the hallmark of excellence *and* accessibility that characterizes the work of the Royal Society of Medicine, this important guide will enable you and your family to gain some control over the way your arthritis is managed, by being better informed.

Peter Richardson
Director of Publications
Royal Society of Medicine

Introduction

This book is aimed at people who, whether or not they have arthritis, want to know more about it. It begins by summarizing the symptoms, moves on to describe the different types of arthritis and then discusses treatment.

The words rheumatism and arthritis are sometimes used interchangeably, as if they mean the same thing. This can be confusing, so to make things clear, I have used the word 'arthritis' in a general sense. To be more specific, inflammatory arthritis includes rheumatoid arthritis and psoriatic arthritis (also known as psoriatic arthropathy). Osteoarthritis is also known as degenerative arthritis (the words osteoarthrosis or osteoarthropathy were previously preferred).

'Rheumatism' is used in a non-specific way to describe symptoms of painful aching in joints and muscles. Older generations rather dreaded the words acute rheumatism, because it meant rheumatic fever. This involved painful joints (arthritis) and fever, but often ended up by damaging the heart. In most western countries this disease is now very rare.

The word 'acute' is used to indicate something happening quite rapidly – coming on over a few hours, days or at the most weeks. In contrast, 'chronic' means something that has been going on for longer: it is not just a description of the severity of the problem. Arthritis that starts acutely can therefore become chronic, but not the other way around.

There are some other words that are also worth explaining at this stage, as they are useful shorthand. Two such words are 'diagnosis' and 'prognosis'. A doctor diagnoses a patient, that is makes a diagnosis of, for example, gout. They may then make a prognosis, meaning a prediction of how the patient will get on.

Another pair of words is 'incidence' and 'prevalence'. The incidence of, for example, back pain, means the frequency with which new cases are observed in a specified group of people or population over any given period of time, such as a year. Prevalence means the total number of cases over a specified period. The incidence of new cases of rheumatoid arthritis is quite low compared with, say, tennis elbow. However, once someone develops rheumatoid arthritis it tends not to clear up, so the accumulation of cases means that the prevalence becomes relatively high compared to tennis elbow.

You may see the word 'syndrome' increasingly often nowadays. This medical term means a pattern of signs and symptoms that are so often found together that they are readily recognizable and are reasonably predictable, but do not amount to a stand-alone disease.

CHAPTER

1

Symptoms and signs of arthritis

Symptoms

The symptoms of arthritis include the following:

- ✧ pain
- ✧ tenderness
- ✧ stiffness
- ✧ swelling
- ✧ weakness
- ✧ fatigue
- ✧ noises and sensations
- ✧ numbness and pins and needles.

Pain

Most patients with arthritis have pain to a greater or lesser degree. The pain of arthritis is made worse by movement. In fact, with the exceptions of gout and septic arthritis, there may be little spontaneous pain unless the joint is moved or

my experience

I really had no idea what having arthritis meant until I developed it about five years ago, in my early 50s. I just started to feel stiff in my knees and around my knuckle joints. I had always been very fit and actually played a lot of football in my teens and into my 20s. So I thought it was just a bit of rheumatism. When it got to the point that I could not do things like climb down ladders without pain in my knees my wife made me see my doctor. My doctor said I had osteoarthritis and I was shocked: I thought that was something that only old retired people got.

pressed. Osteoarthritis is especially characterized by pain associated with weight-bearing and use, such as standing or walking.

Pain is an individual, emotional and subjective feeling, which only the sufferer can truly describe. It generates, and is also influenced by, other emotions such as fear or anxiety as to what it might be caused by. These are reflected in descriptions such as 'unbearable', or 'terrible'.

Tenderness

Tenderness means that pressure produces pain. Inflamed joints are usually tender, but the converse is not necessarily true. Tenderness may not necessarily imply any significant degree of inflammation, but instead may be due to a heightened awareness of pain. This apparent paradox is discussed in Chapter 4.

Stiffness

An arthritic joint often feels stiff as well as painful. Overall stiffness, affecting the whole body and reflecting widespread joint inflammation, is characteristic of inflammatory arthritis: so much so, that a patient's report of the duration of morning stiffness is often used in clinical research studies as a measure of the activity of the arthritis and the response to treatment. Patients with rheumatoid arthritis often stress that the stiffness is more troublesome than the pain.

Swelling

A joint may feel swollen without actually being swollen. However, definite swelling is an

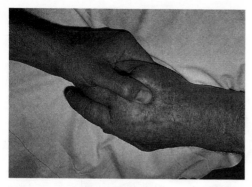

▌Figure 1.1 Hand oedema.

important feature of arthritis. Occasionally, the swelling may involve the whole hand or foot, without being confined to the joints as it is later on in most kinds of arthritis. An example of this sort of swelling, called **oedema**, is shown in the photograph of the puffy hand of a patient, with the thumb of the examining doctor creating a dimple (see figure 1.1). The swelling may be of soft tissue, cartilage, bone or a combination of these. The illustration of a normal joint (figure 1.2) shows the tissues concerned. The swelling that is the most permanent in osteoarthritis is bony. In rheumatoid arthritis the swelling is of the synovial lining and capsule of the joint. It has an almost rubbery consistency. In the group of conditions characterized by **enthesitis** (see Chapter 5) the swelling is at the site of the enthesis. This is the term used to describe the tissue where a tendon or a ligament merges with the bone, near the joint. It may involve the **periosteum**, which is a thin membrane covering all bones, but it is not so clearly confined to the synovium as in rheumatoid arthritis.

oedema
The accumulation of fluid in soft tissue.

enthesitis
The term used to describe the tissue where a ligament, a tendon or a joint capsule merges with or is inserted into a bone.

periosteum
A thin membrane which covers a bone and provides cells that aid healing of fractures.

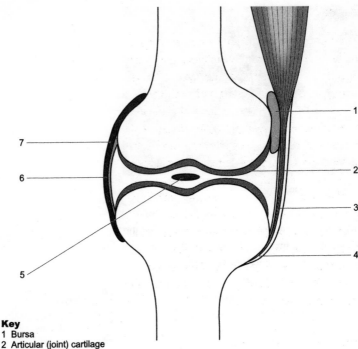

Key
1 Bursa
2 Articular (joint) cartilage
3 Tendon sheath
4 Insertion of tendon (enthesis)
5 Meniscus (cartilage tissue within a joint e.g. the knee meniscus)
6 Synovium (synovial lining of the capsule)
7 Joint capsule surrounding the joint

Figure 1.2 A typical synovial joint.

Weakness

Weakness may mean one of several things. It can be an overall feeling ('I feel so ill and weak'), a real loss of muscle strength (due to nerve damage or muscle disease) or a perception of weakness because of pain, such as in arthritis. Then, the strength of grip may be greatly reduced, without there being anything basically wrong with the muscles: the muscle strength is inhibited, sometimes unconsciously, by the presence of the arthritis.

Fatigue

The fatigue that results from physical exercise is familiar to all, but arthritis sufferers may feel fatigued or exhausted without having done much. Pain itself is exhausting and loss of sleep due to pain even more so. The inflammation characteristic of, for example, active rheumatoid arthritis, is as debilitating as influenza can be. In the condition lupus erythematosus, fatigue may be profound when there is little overt evidence of inflammation; usually, however, there is evidence of abnormality on laboratory testing. Anxiety or depression often cause fatigue: the Chronic Fatigue Syndrome is well known but difficult to define or measure. This aspect is discussed more fully in the section on fibromyalgia – see Chapter 4.

Noises and sensations

Some people can crack their knuckle joints at will, often unnerving others. Those who can do this will know that, once having done so, they have to wait 15 minutes or so before they can do it again. This is thought to be because the cracking noise is due to distraction of the joints, the resulting vacuum causing bubbles of gas to come out of solution in the joint fluid. Time is then required for the fluid to re-dissolve before the joint can be 'cracked' once more. This type of cracking is harmless. However, a different sort of cracking or crackling noise can occur in arthritic joints. This is not necessarily bad news, as the noise bears little relationship to the severity of the arthritis. The exception is a particular type of leathery creaking that is often felt more than heard; this occurs when the cartilage is worn out.

Numbness and pins and needles

These sensations imply an abnormality of a nerve. The 'funny bone' is familiar to most people and is due to a knock on the ulnar nerve as it winds around the inner side of the elbow. A similar painful tingling can occur if the sciatic nerve is irritated at its roots by a bulging disc in the lumbar spine or in the fingers of the hand, as when the median nerve is compressed at the wrist in the carpal tunnel syndrome (see page 45).

A mild numbness or tingling may be felt around arthritic joints – it may be just a slightly altered sensation due to the inflammation. It is not as severe or as predictable as carpal tunnel syndrome.

Colour changes

Part of the process of inflammation is an increase in the blood supply to the affected area or joint. In normal life only some of the microscopic capillary blood vessels in the skin, for example, are opened up to allow blood to flow. Flushing of the cheeks in exertion or embarrassment is a good demonstration of this. In inflammatory arthritis the changes may not be as obvious. Thus, in rheumatoid arthritis the knuckles may just appear a bit bruised, whereas in gout or septic arthritis the whole area is likely to be quite red.

Blood vessels can of course close down as well as open up. Some people always seem to have cold hands. Raynaud's phenomenon means that there is a clear departure from this basically normal situation. All or some of the fingers go white; this is the 'ischaemic' phase, with a visible demarcation from the white to the normal, usually at the bases of the fingers. There is also a 'stasis' phase, where the fingers take on a purplish colour. This phase may be the start of the episode, without an ischaemic phase. The normal circulation will usually finally re-establish itself with a 'reactive hyperaemia' phase, when the blood vessels open up and there is a flush of warmth. Raynaud's phenomenon may be an entirely normal variant, or can be a subtle hint of an impending or underlying connective tissue disorder (see Chapter 7). Cold weather (sometimes even a cold draught), smoking and anxiety are all likely to trigger attacks.

Skin changes are also important in differentiating types of rheumatic disorders, in other words to help make a diagnosis. One example is the skin condition psoriasis. Apart from the changes seen in Raynaud's phenomenon, blood vessels may become inflamed or obstructed by thrombosis, a condition called vasculitis or vasculopathy. This is discussed in Chapter 7.

The weather

Some people do seem to be peculiarly sensitive to changes in the weather. Temperature is the obvious one, but some also have a subtle and rather mysterious awareness of barometric pressure or humidity, as cows must when they lie down if rain is impending. Experimental observations in special laboratories have shown that arthritic symptoms in some people do reflect barometric pressure. There are even websites to help us! (http://www.accuweather.com/)

my experience

I have had rheumatoid arthritis (RA) since I was 35: I am now 40. When it first developed I did not know what was happening. I felt ill, tired and weak. At first I thought I was just run down, because I was working as well as running the household. I put off doing anything about it for ages, but when I found my rings getting so tight I could not get them off I thought I had better do something about it. A friend told me she thought I had arthritis and I should try taking lots of vitamins and to cut out fruits because of the acid in them. However, nothing worked, so I went to my doctor. At first he said he thought it was nothing much, but when the results of the blood tests came back he decided to refer me to the hospital, where they told me I have RA. It took several months to find the right combination of medication for me, and I am left with some permanent swelling and twisting of my fingers and toes, but at least my pain is less. Maybe I have learnt to pace myself better and certainly my family now know they need to help me more around the house, but also I do not feel as tired as I did.

CHAPTER

2

Osteoarthritis

What is osteoarthritis (OA)?

Osteoarthritis (OA) is the commonest form of arthritis. Its frequency rises with age, from being rare below the age of 40, to being evident in most people, to some degree, by the age of 80. However, age is only one of many factors contributing to this almost ubiquitous form of arthritis, which is not really a single disorder. It is partly a description of symptoms and partly of clinical features that can be found on examination. It is also partly a description of what can be seen on X-ray and also what a scientist may find under the microscope.

OA is not regarded as being a type of inflammatory arthritis, despite the name ending in '-itis', which usually denotes inflammation. Alternative names for it are 'osteoarthrosis' or just 'arthrosis'. Often it is just called 'degenerative joint disease'. Some inflammation does occur at

myth
OA is due to age, so the older you get the more you have.

fact
True, but only up to a point. Age is an accumulation of a life time's experiences and actual age in years is only one factor, even if it is the most consistent. So, although almost all elderly people have osteoarthritis, many have no significant problems from it.

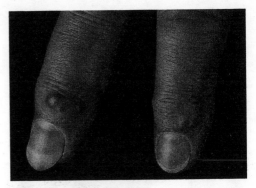

❚ Figure 2.1 The early stages of Heberden's nodes.

various stages in different types of OA. For example, in the hands, the Heberden's nodes that are mentioned below are quite hot and tender when they first appear (see figure 2.1), before they mature into bony outgrowths.

Quite a common complication of OA of the knee and sometimes elsewhere is the shedding of tiny calcium crystals from osteoarthritic cartilage into joint fluid. These produce inflammation which can be so intense that it resembles gout – hence its name 'pseudo-gout'. Its medical term is calcium pyrophosphate deposition disease or CPPD. The patient suffering such an attack may feel ill and feverish. The appearance and symptoms may even raise the suspicion of bacterial infection (which is septic arthritis, see Chapter 8).

Changes

The osteoarthritic process affects any joint tissue (see figure 2.2 where a joint is affected by OA). It affects, at least to some extent, the slippery cartilage of the joint, the bone which is covered

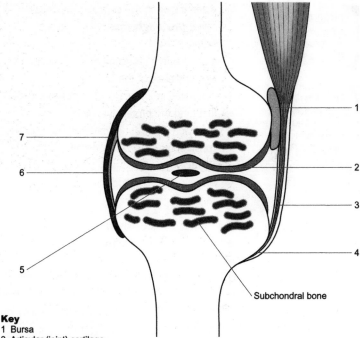

Key
1 Bursa
2 Articular (joint) cartilage
3 Tendon sheath
4 Insertion of tendon (enthesis)
5 Meniscus (cartilage tissue within a joint e.g. the knee meniscus)
6 Synovium (synovial lining of the capsule)
7 Joint capsule surrounding the joint

Figure 2.2 The parts of a joint which may be affected by OA.

by the cartilage and which supports it, the synovial lining membrane and the tough ligamentous joint capsule that surrounds this. The process, however, particularly affects the cartilage covering the joint surface, which normally provides an amazingly slippery articulation. Figure 2.3 shows the difference between normal cartilage and cartilage that is affected by osteoarthritis. These changes caused by OA include the following:

proteoglycans

A chemical component of cartilage that attracts water and swells.

collagen

The main component of connective tissue throughout the body, including cartilage and tendon.

✧ deterioration in the structural chemicals called **proteoglycans**, which attract water

✧ a consequent reduction in the water content and resilience of the cartilage

✧ deterioration in the mesh of **collagen** fibres that bind the proteoglycans

✧ reduction in, or abnormality of, many other constituents such as chondroitin and aggrecan

✧ cracking, fissuring and thinning of the joint cartilage.

The normal cartilage shown in figure 2.3 on the left shows the matrix (the non-cellular meshwork), containing many cartilage cells. The osteoarthritic cartilage shown in figure 2.3 on the right shows the changes, and the resulting alteration in its smoothness and ability to withstand shocks can be imagined.

a) This is a simplified diagram of normal adult cartilage: a resilient mesh of collagen and chemicals such as proteoglycans, which attract water.

b) This is what adult cartilage looks like in osteoarthritis, with deterioration in the collagen and its associated chemicals.

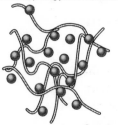 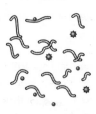

Key

⬤ This represents a molecule of proteoglycan, which tends to swell as it attracts water. The combination with collagen provides resilience to cartilage. As OA develops, proteoglycan function is reduced, and the normal shock-absorbing character of cartilage is lessened.

〜 This represents a fibre of collagen, which provides tensile strength to cartilage. It becomes broken and damaged in OA (see above, right). There are other types of collagen, for example, in skin.

Figure 2.3 Cartilage structure a) normal b) cartilage affected by OA.

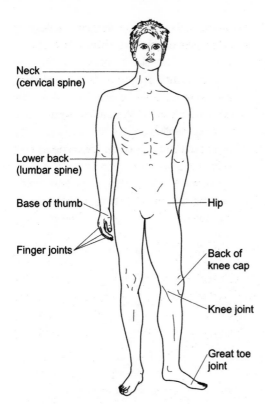

Neck
(cervical spine)

Lower back
(lumbar spine)

Base of thumb

Finger joints

Hip

Back of
knee cap

Knee joint

Great toe
joint

▌ Figure 2.4 Joints most likely to be affected by OA.

These changes do not occur all at the same time or to the same extent. Some joints are much more likely to be affected than others apparently subjected to just as much mechanical stress. Figure 2.4 shows the joints that are most likely to be affected. The ankle joint, for example, is seldom affected by OA unless there has been damage due to recurrent sprains or inflammatory arthritis.

The complexity of the osteoarthritic process explains why there is so much variation in the consequences of OA. One such result is a

Q Can children get OA?

A Children do not develop OA unless they have one of the rare inherited disorders of collagen such as **Stickler syndrome**. However, if a child has a joint that is damaged, for example by infection or a severe fracture, that joint is liable to develop OA in adulthood.

Stickler syndrome
A rare inherited condition of collagen, which results in various degrees of eye problem and a type of premature osteoarthritis.

osteophyte
Bony outgrowth in osteoarthritis.

reduction in the ability of the joint cartilage to withstand a load. As it becomes less able to absorb an impact, like a shock absorber, that shock is transmitted onwards to the underlying bone. So bone is also affected in OA by the changes in structure of the cartilage next to it. In fact, some scientists believe that changes in the bone precede and may cause the changes in the cartilage.

'Wear and tear' is sometimes used to explain OA to patients. It is a term that seems to indicate that old cartilage just wears away. However, the changes in the composition of cartilage that occur with simple ageing are not quite the same as can be identified in osteoarthritis. In fact, the osteoarthritic process is quite active. When changes occur at the level of the molecular structure (the matrix) of joint cartilage, there are compensatory changes elsewhere. So, if the ability of the cartilage to withstand mechanical trauma becomes impaired, there are compensatory changes in the underlying bone, perhaps to spread the load. New but rather abnormal bone grows out at the edge like a buttress: this is called an **osteophyte**. Osteophytes can be felt in their early stages of development and can be seen when they are fully developed. They can often be found at the end joints of the fingers (Heberden's nodes), and at the middle joint of the finger (Bouchard's nodes) – see figure 2.5 – and around the inner junction of the knee joint – see plate 1.

The symptoms of OA include:

◇ pain
◇ stiffness
◇ weakness
◇ grating.

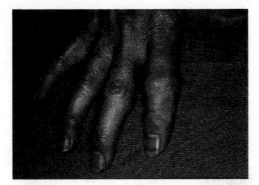

Figure 2.5 Late stages of Heberden's and Bouchard's nodes.

my experience

I am a 55-year-old mother of five children. I remember my mother having very gnarled hands when she was in her 70s, but she still did wonderful tatting and embroidery despite the appearance of her fingers. I started to develop bony bumps at the end joints of my fingers when I was 48. They were very painful as they developed, but the pain has tended to ease up recently, even though I can see that my hands are going to look like my mother's. Unfortunately, I am not as good at embroidery! But at least I can reassure my daughters that they do not need to worry too much.

myth
OA is just 'wear and tear'.

fact
This is partly true. Mechanical stresses do contribute. There is a higher frequency of X-ray evidence of OA in some groups of manual workers. However, just because you can find evidence of OA on an X-ray does not mean that this implies an inevitable health problem.

Pain is the predominant symptom. It may be present as an ache at rest, but gets worse with use. Stiffness is another common symptom: if the arthritic joint is the knee, typically there will be stiffness on first getting up to walk, then it will ease off after a short time. It may worsen with further walking and also with prolonged standing. The site of pain may be at the back of the knee cap (patella), or the inner or the outer side of the joint. A sensation of fullness and pain at the back of the knee may indicate the early accumulation of fluid (effusion) even before the knee becomes appreciably swollen and tight. Such knee effusions are not inevitable; they tend to appear relatively early on in the development of OA, presumably as the function of the synovial lining changes. An effusion may appear later, with substantial inflammation due to the appearance in the fluid of the crystals of calcium pyrophosphate, mentioned above.

Pain may arise from various sites in and around the arthritic joint. The thickened, mildly inflamed capsule is well supplied with nerve fibres capable of transmitting pain. The cartilage itself is probably not so supplied. The underlying bone may be a source of pain.

One form of treatment that was carried out for some years was to 'de-compress' the bone by drilling holes in it, on the basis that pain was due to a raised blood pressure in the veins running through the bone near the joint. The results of this have been equivocal. However, an operation called osteotomy, where the bone near the joint is cut across and the bone allowed to grow together again, can be quite successful at reducing pain although it has largely been superseded. Other potentially painful tissues around the joint include the ligaments and sites of insertion of tendons and bursae. For example, in OA of the knee there is often pain and tenderness around the point at which the capsule of the joint joins the inner aspect of the tibial bone. This is about 3 cm below the joint line, well away from the arthritic process.

Pain is sometimes quite sharp. For example, when the arthritic process is at the base of the thumb (see figure 2.6) it may be so sudden

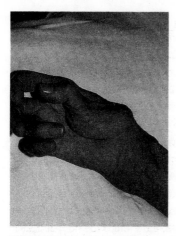

❚ Figure 2.6 Osteoarthritis at the base of the thumb.

that the sufferer cannot help dropping things. When it is at the joint at the base of the great toe, kneeling can produce very severe pain because the toe joint is unable to bend back as normal.

Muscle weakness is one of the problems that is associated with osteoarthritis. The hand grip, for example, is poor partly because of pain, but also because the muscles become weak around any arthritic joint. This is a particular problem around the knee, where the thigh muscles (quadriceps) are a very important component of normal stability.

Grating noises and crackles (the medical term is **crepitus**) are actually rather a poor guide to the severity of the arthritis. We all know people whose joints have always 'cracked'. However, there is a particular rather unsettling and painful crepitus that develops when the cartilage is so thin that bone ends are rubbing together. This is the stage of joint failure.

crepitus
A crunchy noise and sensation within joints or tendons.

Spinal OA

Back pain is covered in a separate publication in this series, but some comments are included here because OA is the cause of much back pain in middle and later life. It is common, say, when a 50-year-old man appears in clinic complaining of stiffness, pain or 'locking' of his back, to find that he can recall, on prompting, an earlier episode of acute back pain and sciatica, maybe in his twenties. Prolapsed (herniated, or 'slipped') disc is really a condition of younger adults. By the time one gets to one's forties the normal discs in the spine have become relatively desiccated (dried). At that stage the central **nucleus pulposum**, which is a bit like the soft centre of a chocolate, can no longer squeeze out through a defect in the outer rim, or **annulus fibrosus**. Sometimes the nucleus will have dried out without the patient recalling much in the way of a history of back or neck pain. Figure 2.7 illustrates a normal spinal vertebra. The vertebrae are a slightly different shape throughout the length of the spine as regards, for instance, the lengths of the bony spinous and lateral processes, but the basic structure is much the same. The close relationship between the disc, the nerve tissue and the small facet joints behind and to the side of the vertebra can be appreciated.

The pictures of a vertebra where there has been a previous disc prolapse (see figures 2.8 and 2.9) show how osteoarthritis has consequently developed, with a narrowing of the affected disc space and a broadening all around the ends of the adjacent vertebral bodies. The new bone intrudes a little into the canal space behind it, where the nerves run downwards.

nucleus pulposum
The centre of intervertebral disc.

annulus fibrosus
The strong rim around each intervertebral disc in the spine.

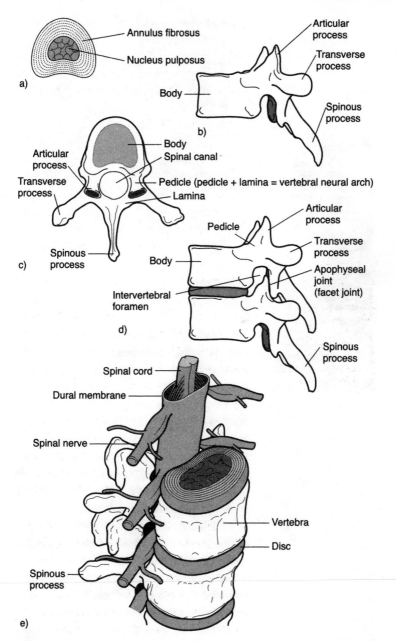

Figure 2.7 A normal spinal vertebra a)–d) thoracic vertebrae e) a lumbar vertebra.

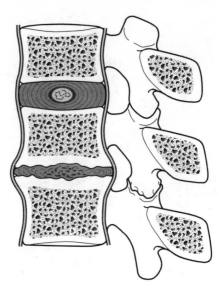

Figure 2.8 The upper disc space is normal; the lower disc space has degenerated.

foramen

The little tunnel or space through which a nerve passes as it emerges from the spine out into the adjacent tissue of nerve bundle e.g. the sciatic nerve.

sciatica

Pain and/or numbness and/or pins and needles radiating from the buttock down the side of the leg to the toes. It is usually not a continuous radiation of pain: there is often a 'gap' of normal sensation down the side of the thigh and knee, with the emphasis being at the side of the calf. This is because the commonest nerve root to be involved is the fifth lumbar nerve root, which supplies sensation to the outer calf.

cruralgia

The equivalent of sciatica, but with pain and numbness at the front of the thigh and knee.

The adjacent facet joint has expanded a little, so that the tunnel (**foramen**) through which the nerve root for that segment of the spine passes, is slightly reduced. This could clearly interfere with the function of that nerve, giving rise to pain or numbness. The symptoms may be just the same as those of a prolapsed disc. If the disc is one of the lower lumbar ones (the fourth or fifth) there will be numbness and pain radiating down the back or outer side of the leg to the toes. This is known as **sciatica**. If the level is a bit higher (third or fourth) the symptoms will be at the front of the thigh and knee, where it is called **cruralgia** rather than sciatica.

If the osteoarthritic process is even more extensive, the osteophytes can be quite large, reducing the ability of the vertebrae to move one upon another, and leading to overall spinal stiffness. This is illustrated in the X-ray of a normal

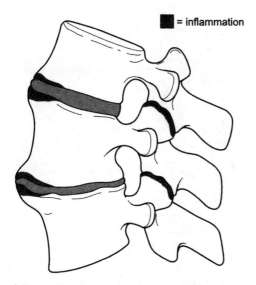

= inflammation

Figure 2.9 A narrowed disc space with osteoarthritis changes at the adjacent facet joint.

lumbar spine alongside one showing advanced lumbar spinal OA, which is termed lumbar **spondylosis** (see plates 2a and b). If the process is even more diffuse and extensive, involving calcification of ligaments as well as the facet joints disc spaces, it has a separate name, diffuse idiopathic skeletal hyperostosis, or DISH. This appearance is also called **Forestier's syndrome**, after the French professor who first described it.

Whatever the medical terminology, the effect on function can be appreciated: stiffness of the spine. Unless there is some interference with nerve function, there is frequently not much pain. The reduction in movement of the back can sometimes be so pronounced that the suspicion is aroused of ankylosing spondylitis (see Chapter 5). Clinically, however, these are usually easily distinguished. Firstly, the patient with ankylosing spondylitis will be in his thirties or forties rather

spondylosis
Osteoarthritis of the spine – especially used in cervical spondylosis (of the neck) or lumbar spondylosis (of the lower back).

Forestier's syndrome
Advanced variant of spinal osteoarthritis.

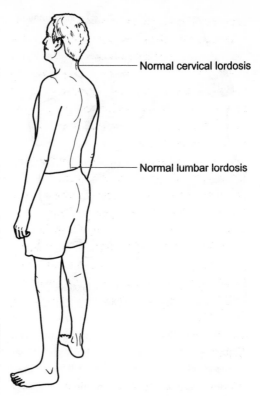

Normal cervical lordosis

Normal lumbar lordosis

Figure 2.10 Normal lordosis of the spine.

than his fifties or sixties; secondly, the patient with ankylosing spondylitis will have a flat lumbar spine, with loss of the normal lumbar curve (**lordosis**) (see figure 2.10), whereas in spondylosis the normal curve is maintained or even exaggerated.

If the space available in the spinal canal for the nerves becomes reduced by osteophytes, the nerve function will be impaired. This causes pain in the legs like sciatica, especially when walking. The pain eases with rest and characteristically by bending forward or

lordosis
Normal inward curve of the spine.

squatting. This symptom of leg pain on walking, called **claudication**, is very similar to the symptoms of **atherosclerosis** of the major blood vessels. The distinction is clear if the leg pulses are normal, but one can have a difficult situation when both conditions are present. The spinal condition is called **spinal stenosis** and usually requires surgery.

So far, the discussion about OA of the spine has focused upon the lower part of the back. The mid-part, the thoracic or dorsal spine, is little affected. The neck (the cervical spine) is affected, if anything, more often than the lumbar spine. Here it is called **cervical spondylosis**. Because the problems associated with cervical spondylosis are so tied up with shoulder and arm rheumatic problems, these are discussed together in Chapter 3.

claudication
Limping, due to poor blood supply.

atherosclerosis
The furring up of arteries that causes heart attacks, strokes or, as used here, pain in the leg.

spinal stenosis
The narrowing of the space for the nerves within the lumbar spine.

cervical spondylosis
Osteoarthritis of the neck.

Causes

We can identify some factors that we know predispose to OA, where it seems very logical that joints may become arthritic because they have been damaged. These include:

⬥ repeated excessive mechanical trauma (e.g. goalkeepers' fingers)
⬥ previous inflammation (e.g. rheumatoid arthritis)
⬥ abnormal joint structure from birth or adolescence (e.g. congenital dislocation of the hip)
⬥ altered joint structure (e.g. OA occurs sooner or later in around half of people following earlier removal of a damaged knee meniscus cartilage).

Q **Is OA more likely in some races than others?**

A It is found all over the world and in all peoples, with some variations. For example, Europeans seem more liable to OA of the hip than other races. This may be due to inheritance or environment.

There are other factors that are linked with OA, but it is not clear exactly how they may lead to the joint damage and changes that are seen. These include:

◇ age
◇ body weight
◇ genetics (especially for certain patterns, such as Heberden's nodes, which tend to affect women)
◇ joint laxity (being hypermobile or 'double-jointed').

As explained above, there is no linear relationship between age and OA. Genes influence the smallest structural components of cartilage, such as collagen or proteoglycans, so there are many ways in which this could lead to OA. However, the anatomical shape of a joint and the body weight of an individual is also partly inherited, so may have an indirect influence on the stresses through the joint. Genes influence the type and nature of the collagen fibres in ligaments, which allow some people to be very flexible and double jointed. This is called hypermobility syndrome and is mentioned again in Chapter 3. Such people have a higher than average likelihood of developing OA at the knee and perhaps elsewhere as well. Maybe this is due to abnormal stresses experienced by the joints, but since the cartilage collagen will be made under the same genetic influence, maybe it is the cartilage that is the problem, rather than the bendiness. Body weight also has a variety of contributory metabolic and behavioural factors that may influence the nature of cartilage.

The causes of OA can therefore be summarized as follows:

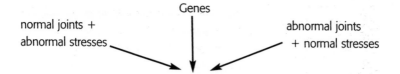

Genes

normal joints +
abnormal stresses

abnormal joints
+ normal stresses

The outcome of OA

The end stage of osteoarthritis is joint failure: when the attempts at natural repair by the processes outlined above are no longer able to compensate for the loads or stresses put upon the damaged joint. This is usually, but not necessarily, also the stage at which pain becomes so severe that surgical salvation is sought. But where the loads are not excessive, such as at the tips of the fingers, the joint may just quietly stiffen up: it has failed as a joint, but nothing needs to be done. In the hip, the pain may settle down but at the cost of losing so much movement that surgery is required to regain reasonably normal function. Similarly, even if the pain settles down as the joint stiffens, it may be at a cost of such loss of function that surgery is required.

Treatment

There is no cure for OA. In the future, new knowledge of the genes involved may lead to ways of preventing it occurring in people who have a severe genetic risk of OA, but at present this is not currently available. Transplantation of healthy cartilage cells into sites of arthritic or traumatic damage has been carried out experimentally and may soon become more widely available. It is also possible that gene therapy, instilling genes for cartilage

Q I know I am somewhat overweight, but all our family are; I feel well and remain very active. Is it true that I risk developing arthritis?

A We know that very overweight people are more likely to develop OA at the knee. We also know that the symptoms of OA can improve in those people when they reduce their weight. So if you do develop knee pain, then losing weight would be sensible, and better than taking tablets for the pain! However, thin people can develop OA too.

development into joints, will reach the stage of clinical practice.

Self-help

The sections above should give all who have been diagnosed with OA some hope that their osteoarthritis need not be crippling. Chronic pain is very disabling, but medication can be troublesome; so anything that one can safely do for oneself is worthwhile considering.

Exercise

This is probably the single most important factor for OA of the weight-bearing joints: the hip and the knee. Normal walking is not going to produce any more damage to an arthritic joint unless it is so near the failure stage anyway that it will not be possible to walk much at all. The muscles, soft tissues and possibly the diseased joint cartilage itself will benefit from exercise. It is not just the joint and muscle tissues themselves that benefit from exercise – it is you. This is a complex subject, and is also touched on in Chapters 4 and 10. Exercise increases the body's output of **endorphins**. These are natural chemical messengers that influence the sensation that we interpret as pain. Intensive exercise causes release of endorphins that contribute to the exultant, satisfying high that many people, not just athletes, feel after physically taxing effort.

endorphins
Body chemicals that help to suppress pain.

Weight

It is also likely that being overweight is a contributing factor to arthritic pain and exercise will be necessary to achieve weight reduction. Weight reduction has been shown to result in less pain in arthritic knees. Aim for your ideal weight. One measure is the Body Mass Index (BMI) which is calculated as the weight (measured in kilograms) divided by the square of your height (measured in metres). Anything over 30 is considered obese: over 40 is morbid obesity. An easier and more practical measure is the waist measurement. If you have an abdominal girth of over 100 cm (39 inches), you are distinctly overweight. This measurement is taken around the fattest part of the tummy, without holding your breath in!

Weight reduction may seem unnecessary unless the arthritic joints are in the hips, knees or feet. However, the other arthritic joints in the spine, shoulders and arms also need exercise and this is easier if you are a normal weight.

Aids

It may be helpful to use walking sticks, which reduce impact loading through the knees. Shoes should have thick shock-absorbing soles. Trainers are good, because they also usually have supportive insoles. Surgical insoles to correct a foot deformity may be helpful for knee pain due to arthritis. A podiatrist would advise on this. Some people find that a knee support helps. Make sure it is not so tight that it digs into the top of the calf as this risks causing pressure on the veins and might lead to thrombosis over time. Physiotherapists may advise a special strapping of the knee cap if it is pulling in an abnormal direction.

Medication

Dietary, herbal and complementary medicine

This is an extensive subject, currently influenced more by opinion than by evidence. There are considerable methodological difficulties in carrying out clinical trials to determine benefit to patients with OA. The selection of patients (hip, knee, hand, spine or a mixture of these) is relevant to the way in which the outcome of treatment is assessed. There are large **placebo** effects, so although subjective reporting by patients is an essential part of such clinical trials, this has to be compensated for by 'blinding', with all the difficulties that implies. X-ray evidence, while being objective, is not of itself necessarily relevant to symptoms. The major problem is lack of a satisfactory end-point for such trials, to determine if the reported benefits are real or imagined. Still, faith in something has its own therapeutic role, so provided no harm results, there are many options worth trying, with little to lose.

placebo
A tablet containing no effective medication.

Glucosamine and Chondroitin

These two substances, derived from a variety of sources such as fish skeleton cartilage, seashells and cow cartilage, are found in the body and certainly have a biological function. Given in tablet or capsule form, they are absorbed to some extent and can be found in blood and joint fluid. They are claimed to relieve the pain of OA. Other claims for their use are that, either separately or together, they restore defects in cartilage and reduce the rate of cartilage degradation. Quite a large number of clinical trials have been carried out with somewhat conflicting results. Overall, there is a reasonable conclusion that there may be some reduction in pain in people suffering from osteoarthritis of the knee. There has also been some evidence that X-ray appearances may improve, but this result could not be reproduced in other studies.

At least these substances appear to be safe. There is a theoretical possibility that since glucosamine is a type of sugar it might upset diabetes control, but this does not seem to be a problem in practice. People allergic to shellfish should find out how the formulation they are considering taking has been derived, as they might react adversely. You should also be aware that the various preparations sold over the counter or by mail order may vary in strength. These are unregulated dietary supplements, so there is less rigorous monitoring of formulation than is applied to pharmaceutical preparations.

Emu oil

This is extracted from the fat off the backs of emus. It has some beneficial anti-inflammatory effects when applied to irritated skin. The claims that it is beneficial when applied to arthritic joints are not well substantiated but it may be helpful.

MSM (methylsulfonylmethane)

This is a breakdown product of dimethylsulfoxide (DMSO), derived from wood pulp, for which many medical claims have been made over the years. Apart from its industrial use as a potent chemical solvent, it is claimed to benefit arthritis and scleroderma (see Chapter 7). It can be smelled, rather unpleasantly, on people who use it. Most doctors are deeply sceptical about it.

Viscosupplementation

Hyaluronic acid, derived from coxcombs or from bacterial culture, is licensed for injection into arthritic joints. In practice, this is confined to the knee. It involves a series of injections directly into the joint, so cannot be described as completely free of risk, any more than steroid injections can. People who are allergic to eggs should avoid products which are made from poultry. After the course of these injections, given over several weeks, pain may be temporarily relieved. However, considering the tendency to variation in OA symptoms, improvement may be due to chance and is certainly not permanent.

Analgesics

Simple analgesics, principally paracetamol or low dose NSAID (ibuprofen), are the basic form of treatment for managing the pain and stiffness of OA. There is good clinical trial evidence that this approach is as effective in most cases and certainly safer than prolonged use of NSAIDs in higher doses. If, however, the latter are necessary, their possible gastrointestinal, kidney and other side-effects must be borne in mind. This topic is also discussed in Chapter 10.

Joint aspiration (removal of fluid)

Synovial fluid effusions ('water on the knee') may require removal to relieve pain and to allow restoration of normal function. This is usually followed by the injection of steroid, as the benefit tends to be longer lasting. It is not a cure for OA, but can certainly give temporary relief. Injection into other sites, such as the hand, elbow or shoulder is carried out when the local symptoms indicate that such an injection is likely to help.

Surgery

There are some helpful conservative operations, such as knee washouts, but here we will focus on surgery to replace a failed joint with an artificial joint. Approximately 30,000 knee replacements and 50,000 hip replacements are carried out in the UK each year and the vast majority of these are for OA. The procedure of hip replacement has probably made more difference to more people's lives than any other elective surgical operation. The success rate for hip replacement is well over 90 per cent. There is, as with any major surgery, a risk of death or serious complication, but these rates have improved to the extent that almost everyone knows of someone who has had a successful hip or knee replacement.

There is a need for caution, however. A non-biological material is being inserted into the body and the materials may not be tolerated, added to which there is always a small but definite risk of infection. The joint, being a mechanical artefact, will eventually wear out. Replacement of an artificial joint with another, a procedure known as revision arthroplasty, carries a lower success rate than the primary procedure. Revision surgery is almost becoming a specialty itself.

Surgery for OA of other joints is more problematical. The range of possible approaches is large and it is not possible to discuss here the individual procedures with their risks and benefits, as they will vary from patient to patient and surgeon to surgeon. There are some principles however. Mostly, surgery is for pain. A surgeon may be successful at reducing or eliminating the pain of an arthritic joint, but the patient must be aware that that joint is not being restored to its normal former self. There may be improvement in the range of motion over the arthritic joint, but it will not be that of a normal one. This is especially worth remembering, for example, where the knee or the base of thumb joint is concerned.

CHAPTER

3

Soft tissue problems

These are extremely common: virtually everyone will have some such trouble, even if only mildly, at one time or another. The conditions include lesions of tendons, **bursae**, ligaments and joints. The following list is not intended to be comprehensive but, for the purposes of this chapter, neck pain and some peripheral nerve problems are included. Mention is also made of two specific abnormalities of soft tissue: hypermobility and Dupuytren's contracture.

bursae
Cushioning sacs over a bony prominence.

Common soft tissue problems

Pain in the neck and arm

Neck pain:

✧ acute wry neck and cervical disc prolapse
✧ whiplash-type injury
✧ cervical spondylosis.

Pain in the shoulder region:

✧ rotator cuff problems
✧ acromio-clavicular joint (ACJ) joint problems
✧ calcific bursitis
✧ frozen shoulder.

Pain in the arm:

✧ tennis elbow
✧ golfer's elbow
✧ forearm pain
✧ olecranon bursitis.

Problems in the wrist and hand

✧ De Quervain's tenosynovitis
✧ ulnar nerve compression
✧ carpal tunnel syndrome
✧ trigger finger
✧ ganglion
✧ Dupuytren's contracture.

Pain in the hip and leg

✧ differential diagnosis
✧ greater trochanteric bursitis
✧ knee bursitis (anserine, patellar).

Problems with the foot

✧ tarsal tunnel
✧ bunion pain
✧ plantar fasciitis and heel spurs
✧ postural pain.

Hypermobility syndrome

This chapter is not intended as a manual for self-diagnosis, but as a guide to the nature of the problems and their prognosis, with and without treatment. Figure 3.1 illustrates the sites of the common soft tissue problems.

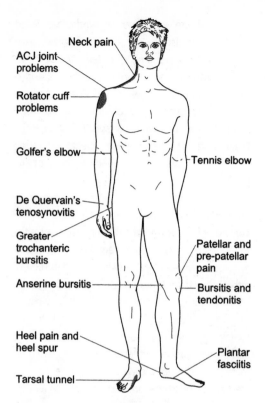

Neck pain

ACJ joint problems

Rotator cuff problems

Golfer's elbow

De Quervain's tenosynovitis

Greater trochanteric bursitis

Anserine bursitis

Heel pain and heel spur

Tarsal tunnel

Tennis elbow

Patellar and pre-patellar pain

Bursitis and tendonitis

Plantar fasciitis

Figure 3.1 Sites of soft tissue rheumatic problems.

Causes

These problems are localized lesions of the tendons, bursae, ligaments or joint capsules. Contributory factors include individual inherent susceptibility (such as hypermobility or Dupuytren's contracture) and mechanical trauma or unaccustomed use. The degree to which one of these problems becomes a disability depends upon a whole set of other factors. These include occupational demands, psychosocial aspects, family and personal support systems and the outcome of prevention or treatment.

Many of the problems or syndromes listed above would also be encompassed by the term 'work-related upper limb disorders' (WRULD) or, by a previously more common term, 'repetitive strain injury' (RSI). However, this does not mean that having one of these problems suggests that it is necessarily related to a specific occupation. Discussion of the wider aspects of such occupational disorders is beyond the scope of this book.

These conditions are not primarily caused by inflammation, except where they arise in the context of a form of inflammatory arthritis. Examples of these include carpal or tarsal tunnel syndrome where the synovitis of inflammatory arthritis, such as rheumatoid arthritis, can cause compression of the median nerve at the wrist or the tarsal nerve at the ankle (tarsal tunnel syndrome). Similarly, plantar fasciitis occurs as a component of the spondylarthropathies, such as Reiter's syndrome. However, there is a definite element of inflammation in all of them, generated by the process of repair of micro-trauma.

Neck pain

Acute wry neck

Acute 'wry neck' can occur in adolescents. In the absence of identifiable considerable trauma, the possibilities of neurological or behavioural abnormalities should be considered. Pain in the neck is an obvious symptom and it tends to be more to one side than on both sides. It may radiate up the back of the head to one side, or over the eyes as a headache. The muscles at the

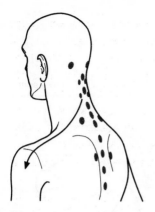

▌Figure 3.2 Sites of radiation of neck pain.

base of the neck are tender if pinched and movement or rotation to one side is usually more restricted than to the other. If there is pain or pins and needles down to the hand, then this usually means that a nerve root is compressed. It is not always appreciated, however, that the pain may be transmitted down between the shoulder blades (see figure 3.2)

Cervical disc prolapse

In adults, a prolapsed intervertebral disc is possible and if there are symptoms suggesting nerve involvement, such as pins and needles or numbness, then the likelihood is high. Investigation with high definition imaging is appropriate and conventional X-rays are clearly necessary if there is any possibility of traumatic fracture. In other cases these images won't be very helpful for diagnosis. However, the finding of an abnormal posture of the spine – straightening out of the normal cervical lordosis (inwards curve) – is useful positive confirmation of muscle spasm (see plate 3).

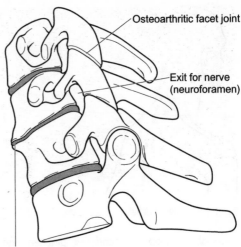

Osteoarthritic facet joint

Exit for nerve
(neuroforamen)

Disc narrowing and bony osteophyte

❚ Figure 3.3 Cervical spondylosis.

Whiplash

The term whiplash is somewhat vexed and has legal implications for compensation claims. There is no definite objective evidence, although occasionally a small chip of bone off the front of a vertebral body is suggestive evidence.

Cervical spondylosis

Cervical spondylosis is osteoarthritis of the cervical spine (see Chapter 2). This involves the soft tissues around the spine and the small facet joints with the development of osteophytes around the discs. The bone changes are shown in figure 3.3 and plate 4. This condition develops in most of the population, starting in the forties, unless there has been an earlier injury or disc prolapse. There may be no particular symptoms,

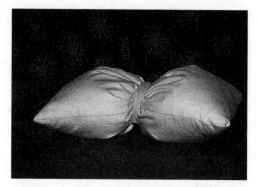

Figure 3.4 A pillow can be adapted to provide neck support.

except for a gradual loss of neck mobility and perhaps some stooping in the sixties or seventies. Other possible symptoms include grinding and dizziness. The intrusion into the exit holes for the nerve roots (see figure 3.3) may result in pain, pins and needles or numbness down one or other arm. Very occasionally this is severe enough to warrant surgical consideration.

Treatment of neck pain

Usually the symptoms settle with pain relief. A surgical collar is often suggested, but do not over-use a collar, or movement can be lost and you risk becoming dependent upon it. A supporting pillow may be helpful and can easily be devised (see figure 3.4). A physiotherapist, chiropractor or osteopath can help the patient regain confidence, show that movement is possible despite pain and that this will settle down as movement is encouraged. If nerve root pain, pins and needles or numbness persist, or become extremely severe despite analgesic tablets, then surgery might be necessary.

my experience

I developed pain in between my shoulder blades after spending a weekend painting ceilings. I couldn't understand how I could have hurt my back that way but the physiotherapist treated my neck and the back pain went away!

Dizziness as a result of neck problems

Pain, pins and needles and numbness are common symptoms of neck problems such as cervical spondylosis. Dizziness is also not an uncommon symptom of neck problems, usually occurring early on and rather temporarily. Balance is mostly achieved through mechanisms in the ear and vision but sensors in the neck also contribute.

Shoulder pain

Rotator cuff problems

The shoulder is a very mobile joint, so has a lax capsule as compared with the hip, for example. It is therefore very dependent upon muscles and ligaments for stability (see figures 3.5 and 3.6). The group of muscles principally involved are the deltoid muscle and the rotator cuff muscles (supraspinatus, infraspinatus and subscapularis). The tendons of these rotator cuff muscles can become frayed and inflamed where they pass under the acromio-clavicular joint (ACJ), which is the junction of the clavicle (collar bone) and the scapula (shoulder blade). This joint becomes

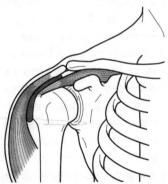

Figure 3.5 Shoulder with arm hanging down.

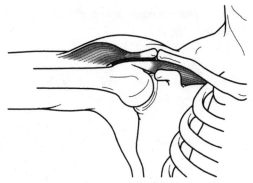

❖ Figure 3.6 Shoulder with arm raised.

arthritic in some people, possibly but not always as a result of many years of heavy manual labour and injuries. More often, in young men, it arises as a result of a sporting injury (e.g. bowling in cricket), weight lifting or a fall on the outstretched arm.

Acromio-clavicular joint problems

The symptoms of shoulder joint, muscle or tendon problems are usually felt in the upper arm. If the tip of the shoulder is where the pain is worst, and if it is made worse on movement, the ACJ or the underlying bursa are more likely to be the problem. If injections of steroid and physiotherapy fail to relieve the pain, a surgical referral will be necessary. Ultrasound diagnosis has proved a real advance in correctly assessing the degree of damage to the cuff tendons and therefore whether a conservative approach will be sufficient.

Calcific bursitis

Calcium crystals can occasionally deposit in the bursa beneath the ACJ (sub-acromial bursa) and

bursitis
Bursitis means inflammation of a bursa, which is a thin double-sided membrane a bit like an uninflated balloon that allows one tissue to glide easily over another. Typically, bursae are situated around bony prominences such as the elbow, knee, shoulder or hip.

this can produce very severe acute pain, like gout (see plate 5).

The shoulder joint does not usually become much of a problem in osteoarthritis, unless it has been injured or the rotator cuff tendons have become very frayed over time.

Frozen shoulder

Frozen shoulder (adhesive capsulitis) is quite a common condition in middle-aged or older people. The onset is usually quite progressive and apparently spontaneous, although injury may precede it. It may involve one or both shoulders, which become very painful, often disturbing sleep. Its cause is uncertain, but there is certainly intense inflammation of the shoulder capsule, which loses all its normal stretchiness. There is an initial inflammatory phase, when the joint feels warm and may be slightly swollen and the pain may be considerable. There follows a 'freezing' phase lasting several months. The shoulder movements are restricted in all directions and dressing becomes difficult.

Subsequently, the slow 'unfreezing' phase takes several months. The whole process lasts 18–24 months and recovery is eventually often surprisingly complete in terms of function. Steroid injections are often given in the belief that it may be a modified rotator cuff problem, but response in frozen shoulder is poor. Sometimes a course of oral steroids is helpful for pain, but usually it is best to stick to pain relief with analgesics. Exercise should be aimed at maintaining the optimum range of movement, rather than stretching inflamed tissue.

Pain in the arm

Tennis and golfer's elbow

Tennis elbow (at the outer aspect of the elbow) is much more common than golfer's elbow (the inner aspect of the elbow). Both result in pain when trying to grip hard. In tennis elbow the tendons of the muscles that extend (bend back) the wrist and straighten the fingers become inflamed and perhaps frayed where they attach to the bone. Usually there is an identifiable cause. This may be an identifiable repetitive over-use such as in sport, or, an unaccustomed activity in someone not used to manual tasks, such as the 'weekend professional'. The problem may settle down with time so long as the sufferer refrains from the culprit activity. If tennis is indeed the problem, then consulting a professional sports therapist is sensible. A tennis elbow 'splint' can also ease the problem even if it is not due to tennis. A steroid injection is helpful (see figure 3.7) but the patient must refrain completely from the precipitating activity (or anything similar) for

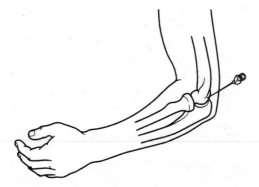

Figure 3.7 The site of an injection to help ease tennis elbow.

two weeks after the injection, or the problem will either not settle or will recur.

Forearm pain

Pain in the region of the elbow that cannot be isolated to a typical site may be due to elbow joint osteoarthritis, in which case the elbow will not straighten fully. Repetitive machinists and keyboard operatives can develop forearm pain that is a mixture of symptoms, often involving tendon and muscle pain, a degree of median nerve compression, and sometimes also interference with other forearm nerves.

The 'funny bone' is actually the ulnar nerve that runs in a groove along the inner aspect of the elbow, where it may be subject to knocks or pressure. In some people it seems to be inherently tight. Pins and needles and pain may be experienced along the inner border of the hand and little finger and surgery is usually required.

Olecranon bursitis

The olecranon bursa, at the tip of the elbow, can become swollen with fluid because of repeated trauma. It may also become infected, and if it is throbbing, tender and red, the fluid should be drawn off and tested for infection. This bursa commonly becomes involved in rheumatoid arthritis and sometimes in gout.

Problems in the wrist and hand

De Quervain's tenosynovitis

The tendon along the upper side of the wrist (holding the hand thumb upwards) may sometimes become inflamed. This is known as de Quervain's tenosynovitis and responds well to a steroid injection and rest.

Carpal tunnel syndrome

Carpal tunnel syndrome is due to pressure on the median nerve. This nerve runs through the wrist to supply the thumb, index, middle and part of the ring finger with a mixture of skin sensation and power (for some of the thumb muscles). The nerve is protected as it runs past the joint by a ligament across the front of the wrist, otherwise it would get damaged frequently. I once saw a bongo drummer who was suffering from carpal tunnel syndrome! An indication of the area in which symptoms are felt is shown in figure 3.8. The pain and numbness or pins and needles are typically worse at night and often the sufferer hangs his or her hand out of bed. It is more common in women and can occur temporarily, but quite severely, during pregnancy. Rheumatoid

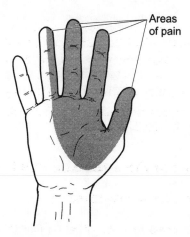

▌Figure 3.8 Areas affected by carpal tunnel syndrome.

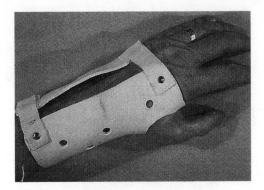

Figure 3.9 A splint used to ease the pain of carpal tunnel syndrome.

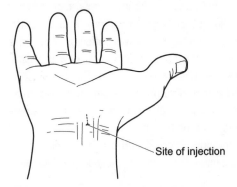

Site of injection

Figure 3.10 Site of carpal tunnel injection.

arthritis also often causes it. A resting splint (see figure 3.9), steroid injection (see figure 3.10), and surgery (see figure 3.11) are usually worth trying in that order and an electrical nerve conduction investigation (EMG) is often carried out to be sure of the diagnosis.

Trigger finger

Trigger finger is due to a thickening on one of the tendons in the palm; the finger (or thumb) gets stuck when bent and straightens with some

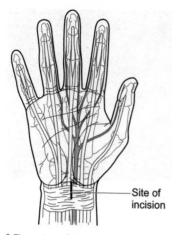
Site of
incision

▌Figure 3.11 Carpal tunnel surgery.

difficulty or not at all. It may occur in rheumatoid arthritis or result from a repetitious task. The nodule can be felt in the palm without difficulty. Usually a steroid injection suffices, but surgery may be needed.

Ganglion

A ganglion is a cystic swelling usually on the back of the wrist. It arises from the wrist joint or one of the sheaths surrounding a tendon. The traditional remedy of thumping it with the family bible is probably a bit out of date for all sorts of reasons! One can put up with it or go for an injection of steroid and local anaesthetic. Surgical removal is straightforward.

Dupuytren's contracture

Dupuytren's contracture is a fibrous contracture of the fascia, which is the tissue beneath and joining to the skin of the palm and fingers. The contracture tends to start at the little finger and

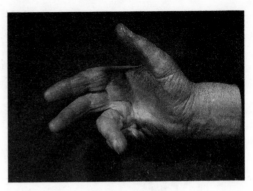

❚ Figure 3.12 Dupuytren's contracture.

progresses to involve the others (see figure 3.12). There is an inherited tendency and there can sometimes be links with other fibrotic conditions such as liver cirrhosis. Surgery usually becomes necessary.

Pain in the hip and leg

Greater trochanteric bursitis

Pain over the hip may be due to arthritis of the hip, or pain radiating from the lower part of the back, or inflammation of the bursa, the cushion that lies over the prominence of the hip (see figure 3.1). This bursa also merges with the **fascia lata**, which is the sheet of musculo-tendinous material passing down the side of the thigh. Alternatively, these three problems can all occur together, especially in overweight people. Hip joint pain itself may be felt in the groin or buttock.

fascia lata
Strong flat ligament down the side of the thigh.

Knee bursitis

Bursitis around the knee has several definite occupational associations which include: carpet layer's knee (see figure 3.13), roofer's knee and

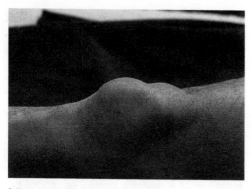

¶ Figure 3.13 Carpet layer's knee.

housemaid's knee. These are basically the same condition, although the actual bursa (there are about a dozen different ones around the knee) may differ. 'Beat knee' was the term used for coal-miners' knee bursitis. Athletes can develop **anserine bursitis** or pre-patellar bursitis associated with over- use or repeated trauma. Tendonitis of the tendon from the patella (knee cap) in an adolescent may closely resemble a condition of adolescence called Osgood-Schlatter's disease. This involves the insertion of the patellar tendon into the tibial bone and is a form of **osteo-chondritis**.

anserine bursitis
This bursa lies at the inner aspect of the knee.

osteo-chondritis
Mild inflammatory condition of growing joints and bones.

Problems with the foot

Feet vary enormously and the different shapes can be seen by the footprints in figure 3.14. Neither a flat foot nor a high arched foot is necessarily painful, although both may be associated with calluses over prominences.

Postural pain

Postural pain can occur if foot posture is very poor: you can see this sometimes by looking at people's feet as they walk and noticing how the heel may turn in or out or if the shoe is badly worn. Some people are amazingly sloppy about their footwear!

Tarsal tunnel

Tarsal tunnel is analogous to carpal tunnel but it occurs in the foot instead of the hand. Just as the median nerve at the wrist is protected by a ligament across the wrist beneath the skin, the tarsal tunnel is where a nerve runs around the inner side of the ankle beneath the bony prominence. The pain is felt along the inner border of the foot. It is not as common as carpal tunnel syndrome and tends to occur in people who already have some form of arthritis in the foot which causes swelling within the tarsal tunnel, affecting the function of the nerve that runs through it.

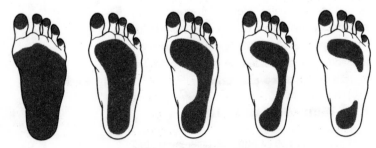

Figure 3.14 Variations in the arch of the foot.

Bunion pain

The commonest arthritic problem in the foot is osteoarthritis (OA) of the great toe joint, the first metatarsal-phalangeal joint. A bunion is a common accompaniment, but is not a pre-requisite, as arthritis of the toe may result in loss

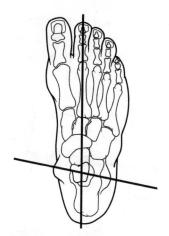

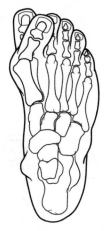

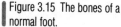
Figure 3.15 The bones of a normal foot.

Figure 3.16 The deformity of a bunion joint.

of movement of the joint with no deformity (hallux rigidus) – see figures 3.15 and 3.16.

Plantar fasciitis and heel spurs

Plantar fasciitis is a painful disorder of the plantar fascia, which is a ligament-like structure that stretches from the heel bone towards the front of the foot (see figure 3.17 and plate 6). It is more common with age, but not necessarily advanced age. It occurs variously as a result of unaccustomed walking or other over-use, such as prolonged standing on step-ladders. It is also common in obesity. It is best treated conservatively by losing weight, if overweight, revising your footwear and by stretching. It is also worth consulting a podiatrist about insoles. Steroid injections have a limited use and surgery hardly ever works. A case has been made for extracorporeal ultra sound shockwave therapy but it is unproven. A heel spur may be blamed. Heel spurs are long outgrowths forming the origin of the plantar fascia. They are quite

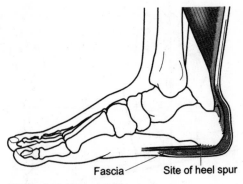

Fascia   Site of heel spur

Figure 3.17 Plantar fasciitis.

normal. There is no proven relationship between the presence of heel spurs and the development of plantar fasciitis, except in certain types of spondylarthropathy, such as psoriatic arthritis or Reiter's syndrome. In these cases the heel spur will be seen on X-ray to be rather indistinct. This is because it is an inflammatory enthesitis, where the fascia meets the spur.

Hypermobility

Hypermobility is difficult to define, since there is no clear distinction between pathological hypermobility and normality, especially in children, where up to 20 to 30 per cent have been said to be hypermobile. A joint has a range of normal movement that is limited by the ligaments and capsule around it. These soft tissues are mostly composed of collagen. Collagen is a large complex molecule, which differs slightly from tissue to tissue (skin, cartilage, tendon, heart etc.). You may inherit a slight variation in your collagen that allows you to be a bit more bendy than average, in which case you are said to be 'double jointed'. There are genetic variations, however, that are more troublesome; one example is Ehlers-Danlos syndrome. Hypermobility syndrome is not a disease but a variant of normal which is associated with certain symptoms. Schemes to enable the classification of joint hypermobility for research purposes are based on a combination of abnormal ranges of motion shown in figures 3.18 to 3.21

A person is not defined as being hypermobile if they can just, for example, bend over to touch their toes – they have to have a 'full house' of bendiness! Ballet dancers and circus contortionists benefit from this innate ability but there is a definite, although not inevitable, association with osteoarthritis. This is clearest in the case of the knee and of the thumb. Aching, joint pain and recurrent knee effusions (fluid accumulation) are all more frequent in hypermobile people. Treatment is aimed at relieving symptoms when necessary. This could be something simple such as heat or an ice pack. A knee effusion may

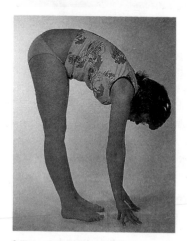

Figure 3.18 Hypermobility 1: fingers to floor.

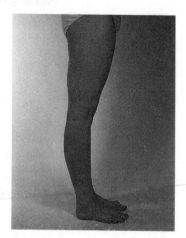

Figure 3.19 Hypermobility 2: hyperextended knees.

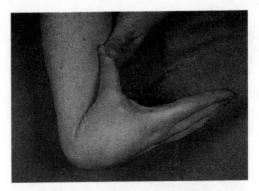

Figure 3.20 Hypermobility 3: thumb to wrist.

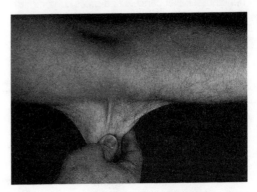

Figure 3.21 Hypermobility 4: skin stretching.

require draining off, or pain-relieving medication might be helpful. More severe inherited abnormalities of collagen, such as Ehlers-Danlos, are associated with excessive laxity of the skin but also abnormalities that may be more serious, such as cardiac or other vascular disorders. Specialist medical opinion is advisable for these conditions.

Hints for reducing work-related rheumatic problems

The following points may help to reduce work-related problems.

Try:

- reducing repetitive tasks
- reducing the risk of unexpected loads
- reducing the amount of force required in carrying out a task
- identifying the most appropriate working position for the individual
- improving the environment at work (including teamwork and communication between staff and employers).

Complex regional pain syndrome

This has also been known as causalgia and also reflex sympathetic dystrophy (RSD). This range of names is an indication of its peculiarities. Very simply (perhaps too simply!) it is a set of symptoms and signs that occur usually in a hand or foot, but can involve a whole arm or leg. The hand (or foot) will be painful and tender, rather dusky in colour and a bit sweaty, yet quite cool to touch. This is because it involves altered function of the sympathetic nerves, which control the blood vessels. The problem may develop after an injury, such as a fracture. It may pass off spontaneously, but once fully developed can be quite difficult to treat and requires referral to a specialist service such as a pain clinic.

Myofascial pain syndromes

This term is sometimes used as a rather grand way of describing non-specific aching tenderness in the upper back, but it also gets interchanged with fibrositis. This term is less often used nowadays; it means localized tender points such as around the shoulder blade. Actual tender nodules can be found and occasionally successfully massaged away, or injected with local anaesthetic to relieve pain and tenderness. When widespread pain and tenderness develops, the term fibro-myalgia is more likely to be used (see Chapter 4).

CHAPTER

4

Fibromyalgia

This is a name given to a group of symptoms, rather than to an established disease. The case history below gives a typical story and has been altered for anonymity.

Case history

Janet is 53 years old. She has tended to suffer from aches and pains for many years, but they have become much worse recently, since her menopause. She aches all over and her arms feel tight and tender. She does not like anyone to put an arm around her shoulders. She gets pins and needles in her hands and up her arms. Her doctor wondered about carpal tunnel syndrome, but electrical tests were negative. She sleeps poorly: she goes off to sleep all right but then wakes up, tosses and turns, goes to the toilet and may then sleep until quite late, but wakes up feeling tired. She is fatigued, irritable and is worried about her memory being poor. Her bowels are a bit irregular and she also passes urine frequently. Her mouth is a bit dry and she drinks water or tea frequently. She feels unable to do things around the house properly.

Here is an outline of what Janet's doctor finds when she comes to the clinic.

> She is a neatly dressed woman, looking despondent and rather tense. She is accompanied by her husband, who is anxious about her. When Janet turns to him for support in explaining her difficulties, he reassures her. He also says to the doctor that he is always telling her to rest and not to try to do too much, but that she is worried about keeping the house tidy.
>
> On examining Janet, the doctor finds she has pain when raising her arms above her shoulders or putting her hands behind her back as if to do up her bra, but that she can actually achieve that, with an effort. There are numerous places where she winces with tenderness on very light touch, such as at the nape of her neck, or around her elbows. Her tummy is tender on light pressure and she says that it feels bloated. She has pain across the lower part of her back. However, she can actually move, with discomfort, reasonably well. The doctor finds slight bony swellings, some of which are a bit tender on squeezing, on several of Janet's fingers. However, there is no evidence of soft tissue swelling of any of her joints.

Janet has fibromyalgia. She has real pain, discomfort, tenderness and disability. When she is examined there is only evidence of minor osteoarthritis in her fingers. The doctor feels confident that there is no inflammation. However, partly to reassure Janet and her husband, some blood tests are carried out and her back and hands are X-rayed. The results of the blood tests show that the haemoglobin level and full blood count are normal. The **ESR** (erythrocyte sedimentation rate) is 14 mm per hour (which is normal) and the rheumatoid factor test is negative. The anti-nuclear antibody (ANA) test is also negative. The X-rays show changes of minor degeneration of the disc between the fourth and fifth lumbar vertebra.

ESR
Erythrocyte sedimentation rate: this measures inflammation, infection or abnormalities in serum proteins.

The results support the doctor's judgement that there is no sign of disease. The ESR, being normal, rules out any significant inflammatory process, but Janet still has pain, discomfort and despondency. She is being told that there is nothing wrong and this makes her feel worse, because no one will now believe that she has these problems. She has a somewhat despairing feeling that everything is being put down to her menopause. How can these troublesome symptoms be explained?

Explanation of symptoms

Fibromyalgia is related to a number of other situations where there is a problem of dysfunction rather than disease; these conditions include restless leg syndrome, irritable bowel syndrome, chronic fatigue syndrome and ME (myalgic encephalomyelitis). As with those conditions, there have been arguments in various media as to whether fibromyalgia exists as what one might call a 'real' disease, with accusations from vociferous sufferers that doctors do not believe their symptoms. This has to some extent been countered by research findings of abnormal nervous and endocrine (hormone) system function in people with fibromyalgia. In turn, this research has been met with some scepticism as not being specific to fibromyalgia, and that these changes can be found in any stressful condition. The term 'abnormal autonomic arousal' syndrome has been coined to describe the findings.

The symptoms of fibromyalgia are quite common in patients with **lupus** and **Sjögren's syndrome** and it is sometimes difficult to distinguish active inflammation from fibromyalgia.

lupus
Short for Systemic Lupus Ergthematosus (SLE). (See Chapter 7 for details.)

Sjögren's syndrome
Where the sufferer has inadequate saliva and tears along with rheumatic and other symptoms. (See Chapter 7.)

However, there is much anxiety associated with the variability of true lupus symptoms, so this is not surprising. The finding of a positive ANA test in a patient with fibromyalgia always presents diagnostic difficulties. A 'whiplash' collision or other similar injury, or a minor back strain, in a patient with fibromyalgia often sets the symptom complex off again.

It is useful to remember that pain is an emotion. It is just as real, but may have no underlying physical cause. Or there may be a cause such as osteoarthritis (OA), with anxiety compounding the symptoms. Some people would latch onto the X-ray findings in the example given, as providing evidence of an underlying spinal problem. Yet such X-ray findings are common and bear virtually no relationship to symptoms. In fact, one can argue that there is no point in X-raying someone's back if the symptoms and examination are reassuring evidence of lack of disease.

An important feature of fibromyalgia is the lack of a normal sleep pattern. Sleeping may seem long enough: the sufferer may wake feeling groggy as if she has slept deeply, but in fact she still feels tired on waking up fully. She may even sleep during the day as well. Her disability may not be very profound to her family: she may appear to be getting on with things as well as ever, so they may not appreciate the difficulties she has in doing what used to be straightforward. She may have rather high ideals about tidiness, for example, and what may appear exemplary to others is less than satisfactory to her, so her suffering may be partly because she feels it is not understood properly. The partners of many patients say to me that the patient has an almost excessively tidy kitchen.

The emphasis so far has been on women. This is because fibromyalgia is predominantly diagnosed in women. It is unusual in men and whether this means that they experience fewer symptoms or just present themselves to doctors less often is not clear. When a male does develop fibromyalgia, the features appear similar to those in women.

How is fibromyalgia diagnosed?

The typical tender areas (shown in figure 4.1) are the only clinical signs and, as may be imagined, are not very objective. They are areas around joints, but not actually at the site of the joint itself. Testing for tenderness is rather subjective: clearly doctors are unlikely to exert precisely the same pressure. Nor are the tender sites predictably consistent. They have, however, proved useful for research into fibromyalgia. Criteria have been developed for diagnosing fibromyalgia by organizations such as the American College of Rheumatology (ACR). These may be considered a bit technical so I have attempted to summarize them below. This is my summary, so should not be used to self-diagnose!

The features of the fibromyalgia syndrome

◇ Widespread aches and pain all over the body together with back pain up and down the spine, lasting for at least three months.

◇ Many excessively tender places, confirmed by the doctor pressing firmly over the skin in a standard way in at least 11 out of 18 tender sites. These characteristic tender sites contrast with others that are not tender in fibromyalgia, such as the forehead.

◇ The excessively tender places are on both

sides of the body and are more or less as follows:

- around the base of the skull
- at the lower neck
- the lower back
- in the muscle of the shoulder
- around the shoulder blade
- on the breastbone
- at the elbow
- around the hip and around the knee.

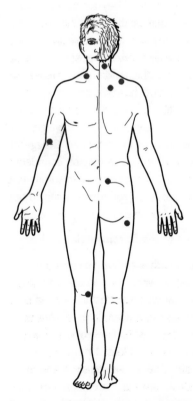

Figure 4.1 The typical tender areas of fibromyalgia.

How is fibromyalgia treated?

The usual pain relief tablets, such as paracetamol or ibuprofen, are less helpful than in, for example, osteoarthritis. If stronger tablets such as codeine are prescribed they are usually no better and may add further uncomfortable side-effects such as grogginess or constipation. Non-steroidal drugs such as diclofenac are unlikely to be any more effective and also run the risk of producing heartburn or indigestion, to which the fibromyalgic patient is already somewhat more liable than average. Powerful pain relievers of the opiate type are clearly quite definitely contra-indicated.

It may be tempting to use sleeping tablets (hypnotics) such as lorazepam or temazepam but these will not necessarily rectify the sleeping problem and are likely to be habit-forming. Herbal remedies (see Chapter 10) may be helpful and preferable alternatives.

In terms of other medicinal treatments, amitryptiline is often recommended. It is a long-established treatment for depression and is helpful for the anxiety that is part of fibromyalgia. It is used in many chronic pain situations, as it seems to help the patient cope with the pain better. However, experience shows that it is best limited to about the first three months in someone with fibromyalgia in order to break the cycle of sleeplessness and fatigue. Past this point dependency creeps in and the benefits wane.

The symptoms of fibromyalgia reflect a self-perpetuating cycle of disquiet, restlessness, anxiety, pain and sleeplessness: a sort of musculoskeletal distress. To break that cycle requires sometimes too much of the individual, and external professional help is needed.

An occupational therapist or physiotherapist has often been the health professional most suited to this but cognitive behavioural therapy (CBT) has also been used with some success. CBT is usually undertaken by a professionally trained clinical psychologist in a hospital or clinic setting. However, this may not be the way that some patients wish to proceed. A supportive but not over-protective family and circle of friends is probably the ideal. Physical exercise is an important component: setting achievable goals for walking or a physical programme is helpful. It is useful to set about this outside of normal everyday activities or family commitments: for example, a set walk or an exercise group. Disciplines such as yoga or t'ai chi, which help with relaxation, are found useful by some people. Pain clinics, provided they offer a behavioural type of approach rather than a medication-led one, may also be helpful.

The personal situation and attitudes of the fibromyalgic sufferer are often at the root of the problem. Previous emotional problems, stress at work or at home, or family discord may contribute but may also be difficult to face up to. Even in consideration of the fact that research shows that there is an abnormal degree of central nervous system 'arousal', an effective treatment plan really should consider a behavioural approach. It is however uncertain how behavioural modification operates and it may be neither acceptable nor effective.

New research indicates that there may be other medications, such as the dopamine agonist drug used in Parkinson's Disease, which may help to normalize the 'arousal' state. However, many doctors feel that this risks reinforcing the perception that people with fibromyalgic symptoms are ill. In other words, to over-medicalize fibromyalgia may be the wrong approach. Fibromyalgia patients have an above-average utilization of all forms of medical care, whether conventional or complementary. Fibromyalgia support groups exist, and mutual sharing of problems and discussion can be very helpful. However, there is also the risk thereby of further reinforcement of fibromyalgia as an 'orphan' disease, one for which the medical profession has no sympathy. As cynics have pointed out, too many doctors can be bad for your health!

CHAPTER

5

Inflammatory arthritis

Q I'm confused: one doctor says I have rheumatoid arthritis, another says no, it is just a type of inflammation of the joints. What is the difference?

A Inflammation can occur in any rheumatic condition, such as bursitis or osteoarthritis, but then it is a secondary process. Inflammatory arthritis means that inflammation is essential to the process. The commonest form is rheumatoid arthritis,

There are three main types of inflammatory arthritis:

1 Rheumatoid arthritis.
2 Spondyloarthropathy group:
   (a) Ankylosing spondylitis
   (b) Psoriatic arthritis
   (c) Colitic arthritis
   (d) Reiter's syndrome
   (e) Colitic arthritis.
3 Arthritis in children.

Rheumatoid arthritis (RA)

Around 300–400,000 people in the UK have rheumatoid arthritis (RA) and of that figure, two-thirds are women. It can start at any age, but usually develops in the forties and fifties. It may develop over a few days, but usually takes several weeks. Once established, it runs a chronic course and rarely clears spontaneously. About 5 per cent of patients develop severe disease with rapidly progressive joint damage. Around 20 per cent always have mild disease, with little significant disability. So most remain prone to continuous joint inflammation, with a risk of joint damage. The earlier this inflammation is suppressed, the less will be the ultimate joint damage and disability and therefore the less likelihood of the patient developing secondary osteoarthritis (OA).

We do not know what starts the process that, once established, we recognize as RA. It must involve something specific to the person, which may be genetic, together with something in the environment. A family history is moderately common but not universal; mother/daughter, sister/sister cases are unusual, even in identical twins. So the children of a mother with RA are far more unlikely to get RA than to get it. Certain genes, from a cluster called HLA DR, account for about one-third of the risk. These genes are involved in immunological reactions. RA is one of a group of conditions called **autoimmune disorders**, which also includes thyroid disease and pernicious anaemia. If the environmental factor were a common infection we would see epidemics of RA, but we do not. Diet might help some patients (see page 78) but no predictably effective special RA diet has been described. Some people suspect modern food additives or environmental toxins, but RA has been around since at least the fourteenth century and is seen all over the world and in all social groups, although with some variation in frequency. For example, in the UK it is more common in the north-west than the south-east.

but sometimes the pattern of symptoms and signs may not be quite typical and one doctor may prefer to 'sit on the fence' before giving it a label. However, treatment can usually start even if the precise pattern has not been established.

autoimmune disorder
When the body's immune system is over-active in certain specific ways, creating abnormally large amounts of antibody proteins, such as Rheumatoid Factor or anti-nucleur antibody, and also specific reactions against the body's own tissues, such as thyroid.

Symptoms

The initial symptoms are pain and stiffness, with reduced function: for example, a weak grip. Some people also feel tired and ill, as if they have a viral infection. Affected joints usually swell, so rings may be need to be removed; or there may be a feeling of tightness behind the knee, with an inability to straighten it. The wrist, knuckle and finger joints are usually affected early on, often symmetrically. The other joints that are commonly involved at one time or another are indicated in figure 5.1.

The inflammation is predominantly 'synovitis'. This word means that there is inflammation of the **synovial membrane** (also called the *synovium*) – see figure 5.2. This synovium lines the joints, the bursae and the sheaths around some tendons. So in addition to joint swelling, these may become swollen or painful, interfering with function, for example, at the shoulder or in the palm. Just as a skin wound may heal with a scar that puckers, so when inflammation in and around joint soft tissue settles, it may be followed by contracture and deformity.

Figure 5.3 shows the left hand of a patient with early RA: people differ, but this is reasonably typical of the changes that can be seen at an early stage. Figure 5.4 shows both hands of a patient with moderately advanced RA.

Inflammation in RA

The inflammation in RA is of two distinct but related types. **Acute inflammation** is the sort with which everyone is familiar. Abrasions, burns or infections are associated with pain, redness (erythema) and swelling. The pain is caused by

synovial membrane
The lining of a joint.

acute inflammation
This may refer to a recent and short-lived reaction to injury, burns or infections and is characterized by pain, tenderness, redness and swelling. In this textual context, it refers to the apparently spontaneous inflammation arising in joints or associated tissues.

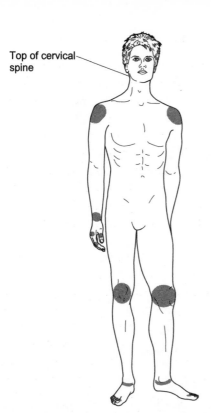

Top of cervical spine

Figure 5.1 Joints commonly involved in rheumatoid arthritis.

chemical messenger proteins; the redness is caused by opening up of blood vessels; and the swelling results from this, with accumulation of tissue fluid. The tiny blood cells involved in this sort of inflammation are white cells called **polymorphonuclear leucocytes**, which non-specifically engulf bacteria, foreign material or tissue debris. It is essentially self-limiting. **Chronic inflammation** arises from persistent activation of the immune system, with involve-ment of other white blood cells, called lympho-cytes. Apart from the troublesome joint swelling

polymorpho-nuclear leucocytes
A sub type of white blood cell – a first-line defence against infection.

chronic inflammation
May look similar to acute inflammation, but long-lasting and with different microscopic features.

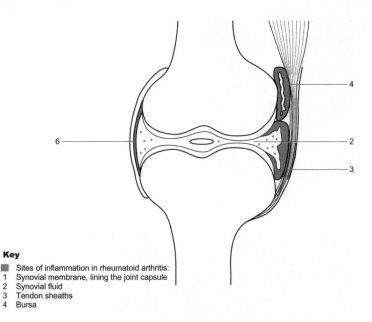

Key

■ Sites of inflammation in rheumatoid arthritis:
1 Synovial membrane, lining the joint capsule
2 Synovial fluid
3 Tendon sheaths
4 Bursa

❚ Figure 5.2 The joint in rheumatoid arthritis.

that constitutes the main manifestation, the most common physical evidence of this immune activation is swelling of the lymphatic glands, for example, in the armpit.

Inflammation in RA may involve other sites, such as blood vessels (**vasculitis**, see page 75). This is similar to, but different from, systemic vasculitis, which is covered in Chapter 7. Various aspects of immune system activation are relevant in all the inflammatory rheumatic disorders. In RA the immune system 'memory cells' produce much larger quantities than normal of an **immunoglobulin** that reacts with other immunoglobulins. This 'autoantibody' is called Rheumatoid Factor and it probably plays a direct role in tissue inflammation. Further

vasculitis

Inflammatory disease of blood vessels.

immunoglobulin

Antibody protein involved in defence against infection but also in chronic immunological conditions.

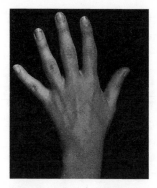

▮ Figure 5.3 Early rheumatoid arthritis.

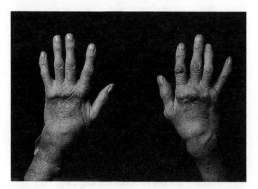

▮ Figure 5.4 Moderately advanced rheumatoid arthritis.

details of these processes are covered in Chapter 11.

If one keeps in mind these two broad pathological processes, acute inflammation and chronic inflammation, it is easier to understand the rationale of treatment. The NSAIDs (e.g. diolofenac or ibuprofen) are effective against acute inflammation, but not chronic inflammation. In contrast, the disease modifying antirheumatic drugs (DMARDs) (e.g. methotrexate) suppress, to a greater or lesser degree, chronic joint inflammation, but do not directly relieve pain or acute inflammation.

tumour necrosis factor (TNF)
A protein involved in inflammation.

Many processes are involved in chronic inflammation, but an important, perhaps crucial, final component is a protein called **tumour necrosis factor (TNF)**. This is one of the many chemical messengers known collectively as cytokines. Although it alone cannot be what causes RA, because it is needed by all of us to defend against infection and other disorders, it seems to be so relevant to chronic synovial inflammation that blocking it is very effective in the majority (not all) of patients with RA. The TNF inhibitors are termed biological agents, often abbreviated to 'biologics'.

This is a very simplistic overview of the problem. There are myriads of unresolved questions about RA.

> **Q** How can the pattern of involvement be explained?
> Why can the arthritis be so remarkably symmetrical, so that the ring finger joints may be identically swollen, but not the index fingers?
> Why are the end joints of the fingers usually spared?
> Why do some patients have much more pain than swelling and some the reverse?
> Why do some patients' joints become very swollen and quite 'floppy', whereas in others the joints just stiffen up?
> Why are some patients' joints cold and clammy whereas others are quite dry and hot?

> **A** Unfortunately there are no answers to these questions; they are not explained by what we currently know of the immune system.

Complications of RA

Complications of RA are much more likely to occur if the condition is not treated successfully at an

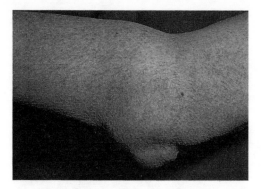

❚ Figure 5.5 Rheumatoid nodules over the elbow.

early stage, before significant joint damage occurs. The term 'rheumatoid disease' is sometimes preferred to rheumatoid arthritis, in order to emphasize that patients may experience problems other than in the joints. This is a brief review:

Nodules

Rheumatoid nodules are little lumps that develop in many patients, mostly over bony points such as the elbow (see figure 5.5). They are almost unique to RA.

Blood and bone marrow problems

The **anaemia of chronic disease** is liable to affect anyone suffering from chronic illness such as inflammation, infection or malignancy. The haemoglobin level falls (i.e. there is anaemia) if there is deficiency of iron in the diet or because of loss of blood (e.g. heavy menstruation). However, in RA the haemoglobin level falls because of the severity of the inflammation, so treatment with iron is unhelpful. It is unusual for the haemoglobin level to fall very far (rarely less than 7 g/litre, which is about half normal) due to inflammation in RA, whereas it may fall much

anaemia of chronic disease
Anaemia due to inflammation or infection, not due to iron deficiency.

lower than that in other forms of anaemia, such as iron deficiency. So if it is very low there is likely to be another or additional cause, such as genuine iron deficiency. The latter may occur because of poor dietary iron intake or because of stomach bleeding due to NSAIDs. Along with the anaemia of active RA goes a rise in the **platelets** and often the **white cell count**.

The **reticulo-endothelial system** consists of the lymphatic glands, the spleen and to some extent the liver. Activation of the immune system by infection or inflammation, as in any inflammatory rheumatic condition, may cause enlargement of these tissues, such as **lymph-adenopathy**. **Haemolytic anaemia** or **Felty's syndrome** are other rare blood complications.

Spinal involvement

The lower spine is not often involved in RA. However, because of the anatomy of the cervical spine (neck) joints, damage to the ligaments stabilizing the neck can become a problem. The symptoms include headache, in some cases weakness or pins and needles in the hands and, rarely nowadays, various forms of paralysis. Surgery is usually required in these situations.

Infection

Septic arthritis may complicate any damaged joint. RA patients can usually notice the difference in symptoms and appearance from the usual arthritic symptoms and urgent antibiotic treatment will be needed (see Chapter 8).

Lung and heart problems

Inflammation of the thin layer of tissue enclosing the lung, the **pleura**, can occur without infection

platelets
Tiny corpuscles involved in clotting.

white cell count
White blood cell count.

reticulo-endothelial system
This is made up of the lymph nodes, the liver, the spleen and the bone marrow.

lymphadenopathy
Enlarged lymph nodes (lymph glands).

haemolytic anaemia
A type of anaemia involving destruction of red cells.

Felty's syndrome
Unusual complication of rheumatoid arthritis, with blood abnormalities.

pleura
The lining around the lungs.

(sterile **pleurisy**). Accumulation of fluid (**pleural effusion**) may accompany this. Rheumatoid **nodules** can grow in the lungs and be mistaken for lung cancer. Lung inflammation (pneumonitis), and scarring (fibrosis) are unusual complications.

The heart is enclosed by the pericardium, a tissue similar to the pleura. **Pericarditis** and **pericardial effusion** are potential complications of active disease and, like pleurisy, can occasionally appear before the arthritis is diagnosed.

It may not be common knowledge that RA carries with it an additional risk of heart attacks and strokes. This is probably due to inflammation itself, above and beyond cigarettes, diabetes or raised blood pressure. So, in addition to receiving treatment for the arthritis, patients should be counselled as regards these aspects of their health. Smoking, in particular, is unwise.

pleurisy
Inflammation of the pleura.

pleural effusion
Fluid in the pleura.

nodules
Little firm swellings found in rheumatoid arthritis.

pericarditis
Inflammation of the sac around the heart.

pericardial effusion
Fluid in the sac around the heart.

Vasculitis

Blood vessel inflammation (vasculitis) may complicate severe RA. It can produce ulceration and other tissue damage, for example to the nerves (see figure 5.6).

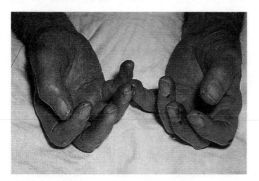

❚ Figure 5.6 Vasculitis in rheumatoid arthritis.

Osteoporosis

osteoporosis
Reduced density of the bones.

Likely causes of **osteoporosis** in RA patients include:

◇ the menopause
◇ steroid treatment
◇ physical inactivity
◇ social isolation and vitamin deficiency
◇ sustained inflammation.

Doctors and patients should be aware of this and take appropriate precautions, which will almost always involve medication. Adequate calcium is essential (and maybe vitamin D) and often a **bisphosphonate** – a drug for treating osteoporosis – is prescribed (see Chapter 9).

bisphosphonate
Drug for treating osteoporosis.

Eye problems

Cataracts can be precipitated by steroid treatment. Dryness of the eyes forms part of Sjögren's syndrome (also see Chapter 7). RA patients may develop a form of this but it can usually be treated effectively with artificial tears. Good dental care is always advisable.

Treatment of patients with RA

The outcome of treating RA depends on the current severity of the arthritis and the outlook for the future (*prognosis*), but also upon the personality, hopes and expectations of the person with the arthritis. For example, there are a few people with RA who, despite quite marked joint inflammation, are able to carry on physical work, ending up with advanced joint damage but little functional restriction. The medical term *typus robustus* has been coined to describe them. There are others whose joints swell little but who are greatly incapacitated by pain.

In terms of treatment, the punishment should fit the crime: meaning that if someone, left untreated, is destined to have a bad outcome then they will usually accept that more potentially risky measures are justified than if their arthritis is to remain mild. To be able to take this stance we need to be able to predict the future and make a prognosis.

Q Can RA be cured? If not, what are the actual aims of treating it?

A In an ideal world, we would understand why a patient gets RA and take away the cause, so curing the condition. However, we are not in that position and the aims of treatment can be summarized as follows:
1 Relief of symptoms
2 Prevention of joint damage
3 Maintenance or restoration of joint function
4 Maintenance or restoration of good morale, independence and social function
5 Maintenance or restoration of overall good health.

General measures

Exercise

Advising patients with RA to rest is of little help: when the arthritis is very active, they cannot do much! However, as soon as pain and weakness permit, normal physical activity and exercise should be resumed, with provisos. A degree of joint protection is best: so if your wrists are swollen, weak and painful, avoid lifting pans or using tools. A physiotherapist or occupational therapist can give detailed advice.

Sleep

If painful joints disturb your sleep, try the following:

✧ Change the timing of pain-relieving medication. For example, paracetamol and ibuprofen are effective for only four to six hours, so if you rely on one or other of these, take it at bedtime. You could discuss with your doctor the possibility of taking a single dose of a long-acting analgesic to take at night.

✧ Stick to a routine: a common cause of insomnia is variation in bedtime.

✧ Avoid caffeinated coffee or tea (or any other stimulant) in the evenings. If you often wake up to go to the toilet, avoid drinking fluid of any sort for two to three hours before bedtime.

✧ Sleeping pills (hypnotic drugs) might be necessary – but try one of the many herbal remedies first (e.g. variations of valerian).

Diet

Diets for arthritis are also discussed in Chapter 10. It is reasonable to postulate that a food constituent could be an environmental trigger for the immune synovitis that characterizes RA. A very few convincing cases have been described where firstly a patient has identified a food constituent which appears to have been responsible for flare-ups and secondly, when the patient excludes that food, the arthritis has gone away. Follow-up of such cases has inevitably been limited, so we do not have clear evidence as regards the permanence of the remission. Exclusion of, for example, dairy products or colouring agents has been claimed more convincingly to be effective in situations such as migraine or irritable bowel syndrome than in RA. If a patient is prepared to keep a detailed diary over several weeks (at least four) of their arthritic symptoms together with the components of their meals, then equally rigorously exclude the suspected item from their diet (again for several weeks), then re-challenge themselves with the said item and keep a record of their symptoms, they might be able to show convincingly that a specific food item is responsible for their symptoms. They should also be congratulated on their diligence – but pity a partner who has to share the diet!

Uncontrolled RA is often a debilitating condition itself, but there is also the possibility of loss of appetite due to feeling ill or drug toxicity and this can result in vitamin or other nutritional deficiencies, so vitamin supplements may be needed to help combat these, as part of a good balanced diet. RA patients are prone to osteoporosis (see Chapter 9). This is due to a combination of factors such as inflammation and relative immobility. Calcium and vitamin D supplementation are advisable in all RA patients if dietary intake of these is poor. Treatment with corticosteroids increases the risk of osteoporosis and subsequently, additional treatment is usually given by means of a bisphosphonate, rather than just vitamin D and calcium.

Body weight

Excess body weight makes life even more uncomfortable for arthritic patients and RA is no exception. Obese patients are strongly advised to reduce their body weight to the average range for the population (see Chapter 10).

> **Q** **What are the warning signs that the arthritis is going to be severe or to be difficult to treat?**
>
> **A** At the present time the following factors, if present over the first few months of the disease, predict a poor outcome (persistent inflammation, joint damage and deformity), if the disease is left untreated:
>
> 1 widespread, persistent synovitis (joint swelling): i.e. once it has started, there is inexorable progression, with little alleviation
> 2 high blood levels of Rheumatoid Factor (a newer antibody test, anti-CCP, is also being increasingly used).
> 3 high levels of inflammatory markers (ESR, CRP – see below) (see Chapter 11)
> 4 persisting anaemia of chronic disease.
>
> However, crystal ball-gazing is not absolutely specific for the individual. Certain genetic markers may predict for liability to severity, but are not specific enough yet.

Who looks after RA patients?

The rheumatology team

People with mild RA may be quite satisfactorily looked after by their doctor. However, persistently active arthritis (joint swelling, raised ESR – erythrocyte sedimentation rate – or **CRP**, stiffness and pain) carries with it the risk of longer term, irreversible, joint damage and other complications. Referral to a rheumatology department or clinic is usually advisable. This is not to exclude the doctor directly seeking the help of therapists for specific problems, but the therapists who spend their time concentrating on arthritis patients are more likely to be able to provide answers or solutions.

CRP
C-reactive protein: part of the infection defence system. This rises rapidly with infection and many types of inflammation.

The occupational therapist (OT)

The OT will:

✧ assess the patient individually in terms of their everyday needs

✧ suggest modified activities to protect
  inflamed joints from undue mechanical
  strain, which might lead to traumatic damage
✧ provide splints to support inflamed or painful
  joints
✧ assess postural or functional demands
  e.g. for keyboard work and household tasks
✧ discuss with the patient the ways in which
  he or she can retain maximum
  independence, including the inevitable
  psychological problems associated with
  disability and dependency.

The physiotherapist (P/T)

The P/T will:

✧ help to reduce pain and swelling with physical
  modalities such as ice, heat or ultrasound
✧ advise on exercise regimens to maintain
  muscle and joint function
✧ advise on pain management
✧ provide splints to aid rehabilitation
✧ provide hydrotherapy programmes when
  appropriate.

The podiatrist

The podiatrist will:

✧ give footwear advice
✧ provide insoles
✧ prevent or treat foot problems such as
  pressure calluses
✧ carry out surgical procedures such as
  osteotomy or bunion removal.

Podiatry is the preferred term to chiropody, in
order to recognize this increasing extension of
their role in specialist care for arthritis.

The rheumatology nurse practitioner

As with the therapists, the nursing role in rheumatology is extending into specialist care. They are essential to the safe supervision of treatment with DMARDs, mostly, but not exclusively in the treatment of inflammatory arthritis.

Pharmacists contribute greatly to the safe care of patients with complex medication. Other health care practitioners, such as radiographers, are at various times also involved in the care of patients with arthritis.

Medical staff

✧ The physician: Rheumatology is a medical sub-speciality, like cardiology or neurology, and so has its own consultants and trainees.

✧ The surgeon: RA patients may be referred, usually by their rheumatologist, for consideration of reconstruction or replacement of a damaged joint. Arthritis surgeons are usually orthopaedic surgeons, who may concentrate on, for example, the lower or upper limbs. Neurosurgeons or plastic surgeons may also sub-specialize in spinal or hand surgery for arthritis.

Medication and the team approach

The drugs used most often nowadays are:

✧ analgesics (painkillers)

✧ non-steroidal anti-inflammatory drugs (NSAIDs). There are many, including ibuprofen, naproxen, meloxicam, piroxicam and diclofenac. They are also marketed under many different trade names.

✧ disease modifying anti-rheumatic drugs (DMARDs):

- Sulfasalazine
- Methotrexate
- Leflunomide
- Hydroxychloroquine
- Ciclosporin (formerly called cyclosporine)
- Myocrisin or one of the other gold salt formulations
- D-penicillamine (rarely, nowadays)
- ✧ cortico-steroids (prednisolone, prednisone, methylprednisolone)
- ✧ immunosuppressives
  - Azathioprine
  - Cyclophosphamide
- ✧ biological therapies
  - anti-TNF (etanercept, infliximab, adalimumab)
  - anti-iL1ra (anakinra)
  - anti-B cell antibody (rituximab).

Analgesia is discussed in Chapter 10. NSAIDs have been the starting point for treating RA for many years and are still beneficial for many patients. However, nowadays we recognize the importance of suppressing the synovitis of RA early in the disease, for the long-term health of the patient as well as the functional integrity of the joints themselves. NSAIDs, despite their name, are usually inadequate for anything other than very mild disease, as they do not, in normally used doses, prevent joint damage. Hence, we use the term 'disease modifying anti-rheumatic drugs' (DMARDs) to cover those drugs that can prevent joint damage and modify the outcome of the disease. These drugs are related only through their effects, rather than their structure. There are some common traits, however, such as slow onset and the need for monitoring for side-effects.

Anyone taking any medication should get to know its name and possible adverse effects. I cannot provide here a comprehensive list.

Sulfasalazine (previously known in the UK as sulphasalazine) was designed in the 1940s as a drug for RA. The original idea, of an aspirin-related compound bound together with an anti-bacterial sulphonamide, was based on the theory that 'focal infection' underlay RA. We do not really know how it works, but probably not through any direct anti-bacterial action. It was the 1970s before sulfasalazine finally found its place for arthritis, although it had been used from the 1950s for inflammatory bowel disease.

As with most DMARDs, a 'start low, go slow' policy is preferred, so the dose is progressively increased over several weeks to a maintenance level. It is relatively well tolerated but if a patient is destined to develop side-effects, it is likely to be in the first six months or so of treatment, during which time the blood is checked about every month for unusual 'silent' side-effects such as liver function disturbance or a low white cell count. About one fifth of patients cannot tolerate an effective dose because of nausea, headaches or general unwellness. A few patients develop more serious intolerance, with rash and fever.

Methotrexate was originally used only in cancer treatment, in much higher doses than for arthritis. If sulfasalazine is ineffective or poorly tolerated, methotrexate is usually the next choice although it may be the first choice in some cases. It is taken usually once a week and is available in tablets of 2.5 mgm and also 10 mgm (it is very important not to mix these up!) and also as an injection, which is sometimes better tolerated.

Second line or 'reserve' drugs

Leflunomide has rather a high frequency of uncomfortable side-effects, especially diarrhoea. However, it is found helpful by some RA patients.

Hydroxychloroquine is also helpful for a small minority, usually in combination with other drugs. It is well tolerated, but it accumulates in pigmented tissue and prolonged use or excess dosage may carry a risk of damage to the retina of the eye. This risk is less than with its forebear, chloroquine, which is rarely used now. Both drugs were originally used for the treatment or prevention of malaria (see also Chapter 7).

Ciclosporin is an immunosuppressive drug that has a small but useful place for treating some patients with RA, although it requires careful monitoring. Cytotoxic drugs such as azathioprine and cyclophosphamide are mostly reserved for diseases such as Lupus, but are occasionally needed for RA. As with the previous drugs, close monitoring is required.

Steroids

Cortico-steroids is the better term, to avoid confusion with body building steroids! Prednisolone and the other forms are very effective at suppressing inflammation. However, doses above 5–10 mgm each day for more than a few weeks are very liable to produce side-effects such as bruising, diabetes, osteoporosis or raised blood pressure. They can also be quite upsetting by producing insomnia or agitation.

Combinations

Taking a combination of DMARDs, such as methotrexate, sulfasalazine and prednisolone, is often more effective and no more risky than using a single drug.

'The biologics'

In recent years the treatment of RA has been transformed by the introduction of biologically produced inhibitors of inflammatory proteins. TNF (tumour necrosis factor) has been identified, to date, as the most pivotal of these mediators of inflammation. It is present, together with another important protein, Interleukin-1, at the sites of inflammation in the synovium, joint fluid and also in the circulation of patients with active disease. Inhibition of this protein with specially produced antibodies or with innate biological inhibitor proteins drastically suppresses inflammation. In the UK, the National Institute for Health and Clinical Excellence (NICE) has approved treatment of RA patients with anti-TNF drugs (including Etanercept, Infliximab and Adalimumab). There are guidelines for using these very expensive drugs, including the requirement for treatment to have failed with conventional regimes of DMARDs as outlined above. These guidelines will be reviewed from time to time. The British Society for Rheumatology has a comprehensive register of patients being treated with these drugs, so as to accumulate the best possible information about their use, effectiveness and side-effects.

An increasing number of patients with other forms of inflammatory arthritis are being considered for treatment with anti-TNF drugs. It seems likely that NICE will issue guidance on this development in the near future.

Any patient being considered for such treatment should discuss the pros and cons with their rheumatology team. These drugs have proved extremely effective, but not in all patients. In view of what is known of the biology of RA, it is not clear why some people do not respond, so more is yet to emerge from research in this field.

Rituximab is an antibody to B cells. These are lymphocyte cells that have a 'memory' of making antibody. This may include the ability to make Rheumatoid Factor, which is itself a type of antibody and may be directly contributing to the inflammation of synovitis. This is a different approach from suppressing TNF with the drugs mentioned above, like infliximab. There have been some recent trials that indicate that this anti-B cell strategy is another potentially useful biological treatment for patients with RA.

The spondylarthropathies

The following conditions are included under this umbrella term:

✧ ankylosing spondylitis (AS)
✧ psoriatic arthritis
✧ Reiter's syndrome
✧ colitic (or enteropathic) arthritis.

Inflammation in the spondylarthropathies

The conditions deserve separate names because they develop in different ways. In contrast to RA, where the main focus is in the synovium that lines most joints, other than the ones throughout the spine, the principal mischief in spondylarthropathy lies in the **enthesis**. Inflammation is therefore called enthesitis or enthesopathy – the 'pathy' bit implies that the degree of actual inflammation is uncertain, but that there is something abnormal there. An enthesis is the junction or insertion of a ligament or tendon into bone. The synovium (the lining membrane) of the

enthesis
The junction or insertion of a ligament or tendon into bone.

knee joints, for example, does sometimes become involved, but much less frequently than in RA. The appearance is different and the joints are rarely involved symmetrically as in RA (see figure 5.7). The hands are hardly ever involved in AS.

Examples of enthesitis:

✧ at the insertion of the Achilles tendon into the back of the heel
✧ sacroiliitis: inflammation of the sacroiliac joints. These large, ligamentous joints are at the base of the spine, linking it with the pelvis (see figure 5.8).
✧ inflammation of the longitudinal ligaments of the spine, leading to fusion of the adjacent vertebrae. When this happens in ankylosing spondylitis it is called 'bamboo spine' (see figure 5.9).

Key

The site of the principal inflammation in the spondylarthropathies: the enthesis. This is the junction of a tendon or ligament with bone. There is less inflammation in the synovium than RA.

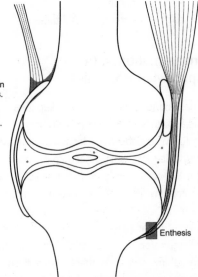

Enthesis

❚ Figure 5.7 A joint in ankylosing spondylitis.

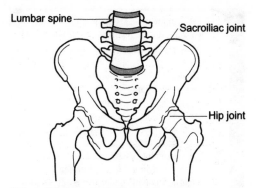

Lumbar spine

Sacroiliac joint

Hip joint

Figure 5.8 Normal sacroiliac joints.

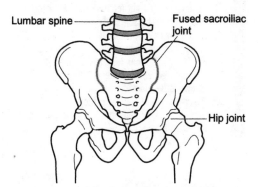

Lumbar spine

Fused sacroiliac joint

Hip joint

Figure 5.9 Fused sacroiliac joints in ankylosing spondylitis.

Q **What is the difference between the spondylarthropathies and RA?**

A The features that are characteristic of spondylarthropathies in general can be summarized as follows:

1   Enthesitis is typical.
2   Stiffening up (ankylosis) of the joints in spondylarthropathies is common.
3   The spine (hence spondyl-) tends to be more involved than peripheral joints – but not exclusively.

A 4   If the peripheral joints are involved, the arthritis is usually not symmetrical, as it is in RA.

5   There is a characteristic appearance of fingers or toes called dactylitis, descriptively called 'sausage toe' or 'sausage finger', which is hardly ever seen in RA.

6   Men are more likely to develop AS than women and are usually more severely affected.

7   The onset of most cases is in early adulthood, rather than middle age.

8   The Rheumatoid Factor blood test that is usually positive in RA is negative in spondylarthropathies – hence the common term 'seronegative arthritis'.

9   There are common links with the skin (psoriasis), the gut (colitis), the eye (iritis) or the urogenital tract (**balanitis**).

10   It is likely that at least some of this group of conditions might be due in an indirect way to bacterial infections (e.g. of the gut).

11   Different genes are involved: the most well-known is B27 in AS.

12   The response of spondylarthropathies to treatment, especially to exercise, is somewhat different from RA.

balanitis
Inflammation or infection of the end of the penis.

Ankylosing spondylitis (AS)

Back pain is very common in the population, affecting around one fifth of us at any one time (see *Your Guide to Back Pain* in this series). AS is an uncommon cause of acute back pain but must be considered as a possible cause of chronic back problems, especially in younger patients. It is a form of inflammatory arthritis that particularly affects the spine. The characteristic aspect of AS is stiffness of the spine, where the lumbar spine has lost its usual curve when the person bends forward (flexes forward).

One of the earliest signs that someone has AS, rather than simple back pain or a slipped disc, is that the ability to bend sideways is reduced in both directions, often without much pain. This is different from simple back pain or back pain due to a prolapsed disc; it is, however, superficially similar to the back pain in middle aged or older people of lumbar spondylosis, which is osteo-arthritis of the facet joints of the spine.

Another difference between AS and 'mechanical' causes is the response to exercise: an AS patient is quite likely to find that exercise is beneficial for back stiffness. The spinal vertebrae are joined together by ligaments, all of which form entheses where they merge with bone and, since the sacroiliac joints are the biggest entheses in the spine, this is where changes of AS are always found. These joints move very little except in pregnancy or very supple (hypermobile) people, so it takes a skilled examiner to notice if that movement has been lost. Even then, it is not always easy to tell if back pain comes from one or both sacroiliac joints. An X-ray or bone scan may reveal changes of inflammation. The ribs joining the breastbone (sternum) can also become inflamed and painful, so odd chest pains are quite common in AS and sometimes need differentiating from heart disease.

Q I am a 30-year-old woman and I have recently developed back pain. I have been told I have a slipped disc, but I have read about AS and I worry that I might have it. How would I tell the difference from back pain due to a strain?

A Men are affected by AS much more than women. Nevertheless, women can get it, so it is quite reasonable to question your diagnosis. Early AS can occasionally resemble a slipped disc, even with some pain in the leg like sciatica, but

A clinical examination will usually quickly distinguish them. We try to avoid X-raying anyone's back, especially young women, but if AS really is suspected, then an X-ray of the pelvis may be required. Blood tests are helpful too: the tests for inflammation (ESR or CRP) in ordinary simple low back pain or disc problems are normal. So if they are raised, one should suspect some other cause, such as AS.

Other problems that might develop in AS

Spinal fracture

The main effects of AS are on the spine. In very advanced AS, rigidity makes the spine more susceptible to fracture than normal. In addition, the vertebral bone structure may become osteoporotic due to the inflammation.

Iritis

This is inflammation of the iris, which gives the colour of the eye, around the pupil; it is part of the uveal tract that lies at the front of the eye (hence also *uveitis*). Iritis rarely affects both eyes, unlike conjunctivitis. The iris is a muscle that widens or contracts to give a smaller or larger pupil. So if it is inflamed, it will be painful to look at light (photophobia) and the conjunctiva (the white part of the eye) may be slightly red. Sjögren's syndrome (dryness) is not found in any of the spondylarthropathies, in contrast to RA or the other connective tissue disorders.

The heart

Rarely, the aortic valve of the heart can become inflamed and leaky.

Lungs

Fibrosis in the upper parts of the lungs is occasionally found on X-ray, but rarely leads to any problems.

The kidney

After many years of active AS, the kidney can very occasionally become affected by amyloidosis, which are deposits of protein. It is detected quite easily by testing for excess protein in the urine.

The skin

Psoriasis seems to accompany AS more often than one would expect by chance, but its management is no different. Likewise, bowel inflammation (Crohn's disease or ulcerative colitis) also seems to occur more frequently than one might expect. There may be common precipitating causes such as infection. Management of the AS is not significantly altered by the unfortunate coincidence.

Genetics and the spondylarthropathies

Inherited factors are important in all the spondylarthropathies, but particularly so in AS. Absolutely everyone with AS carries the gene HLA B27. However, this gene is found in around 7 per cent of the UK population – about 3.5 million people. Since only around 150,000 people in the UK have AS, testing for B27 in patients with back pain has very little value in diagnosis. A patient with AS might worry if they have passed the condition on to a child and may therefore ask for a B27 test to be done. Remember, however, that the B27 is inherited like any other gene, so finding

B27 in the offspring of an AS patient is predictable. It could actually only be of value to exclude AS: but also remember that laboratory tests can be fallible!

Clearly B27 is only a risk factor, requiring some other trigger to set off the condition. We do not know what that trigger is, although bacterial infection is a possibility, by analogy with Reiter's syndrome, where B27 is a risk factor along with the infective trigger. In psoriatic arthritis, the genetic components are less clear-cut, as several different genes play a role in psoriasis itself, with others influencing the expression of arthritis.

Management of AS

The principles of management of a patient with AS are regular daily exercises, with the aid of NSAIDs to relieve stiffness and pain. Failing that, in active disease, treatment with one of the anti-TNF drugs may be appropriate (see above for RA).

Physiotherapy is useful, especially early on in the condition to demonstrate the importance of diligent exercise. This may not prevent stiffening of the spine, but will help to preserve good posture. Occasionally, hip involvement will require treatment by surgical hip replacement. Rarely, surgery to other joints such as the knee or the neck is required

Psoriatic arthritis (PsA)

Psoriasis is a very common skin complaint, affecting around 1 per cent of the UK population, so that arthritis, such as OA, may be coincidental. However, about 10 per cent develop inflammatory arthritis, of which there are several types:

✧ predilection for the small joints at the ends of the fingers (distal inter-phalangeal joints)

✧ psoriatic polyarthritis, with dactylitis or 'sausage finger'

✧ arthritis mutilans: so-called because the finger joints become eroded away and fuse together, leaving no movement at the affected joints

✧ psoriatic spondylitis: which is very similar to AS. The B27 gene is also associated with it. It is often more patchy, with just localized areas of bony outgrowths called syndesmophytes.

crawling around low areas and I do have to take diclofenac, but on the whole I manage very well. I do not know of anyone else in the family who has AS, but my sister has had two attacks of eye inflammation, which I understand is somehow related. I have two teenage sons and a daughter, but they are fit and well.

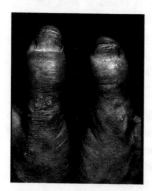

Figure 5.10 A thumb in psoriatic arthritis showing arthritis, psoriasis and nail change.

Treatment of PsA

This is basically very similar to that of RA. If only a small number of joints are significantly affected, local steroid injections and NSAIDs may be sufficient, but if DMARDs are required, methotrexate is quite effective. Biological agents such as the anti-TNF drugs show great promise and many patients are already benefiting, both in terms of their skin and their joints.

Reiter's syndrome

Reiter's syndrome fits into this group because it features enthesitis and also occasionally skin lesions that resemble psoriasis. It is also called 'reactive arthritis', meaning that it occurs as a reaction to infection. This may be of the bowel (certain strains of Shigella or Salmonella dysentery) or the genitourinary tract (non-gonococcal urethritis, usually Chlamydia). It affects individuals genetically predisposed by having the B27 gene. It is not common, but large outbreaks of dysentery have sometimes produced many patients with Reiter's syndrome over a short period of time. Certainly, inflammatory arthritis in young people should always raise the suspicion of Reiter's syndrome, even if the characteristic features are not all present.

Features of Reiter's syndrome (reactive arthritis) include:

✧ arthritis: (tends to be an oligoarthritis, i.e. of a few joints only and tends to affect the lower limb joints e.g. knee, ankle, toes); sacroiliitis
✧ urethritis; balanitis; cervicitis; cystitis; haematuria; hydronephrosis
✧ dysentery: Shigella or Salmonella (certain strains only)
✧ skin and mouth: keratoderma blenorrhagica (looks like psoriasis on the soles or palms); nail problems; mouth ulcers
✧ eyes: conjunctivitis; uveitis
✧ heart: aortic valve problems; heart block.

Outlook for patients with Reiter's syndrome

On the whole, Reiter's syndrome is rather more likely to clear up eventually compared to RA, AS or perhaps PsA, but it may still give rise to continuing symptoms for many months and in some cases years.

Treatment of Reiter's syndrome

Treatment of the arthritis follows the same principles as for PsA. However, because Reiter's can be quite acute and involve systemic complications, as mentioned above, recourse to steroid tablets is more frequent than for PsA. Antibiotics may be administered if there is a proven infection such as Shigella dysentery. Experience with anti-TNF drugs is very limited, because of the relative rarity of patients with chronic Reiter's.

Colitic arthritis

Crohn's disease and ulcerative colitis are types of inflammatory bowel disease. The arthritis that sometimes complicates these conditions tends to affect a relatively small number of joints, often the knees. Flares of the arthritis tend to reflect the degree of bowel inflammation. Conversely, if the colitis is inactive, due to treatment or natural remission, the arthritis will tend to be less troublesome. Knee effusions and ankle or foot problems predominate and joint injections are quite often required for the arthritis. Oral steroids are frequently used for colitis, often in courses at higher doses than are used, for example, in the treatment of RA.

Inflammatory bowel disease may also coincide with AS (see above). Once more, the B27 gene is involved.

Arthritis in children

This section of the book is quite short. This is not a reflection of the relative importance of arthritis

Point to remember
Acute joint infection is an emergency and in this case the child should be seen by an orthopaedic surgeon or rheumatologist the same day.

Point to remember
Any child with suspected arthritis should be seen by a paediatrician or paediatric rheumatologist. The combination of fever, irritability, skin rash and painful swollen joints always raises the possibility of one of the forms of juvenile arthritis.

Point to remember
A medical thermometer is an essential household item: with the knowledge of how to use it and how to interpret the result.

in children compared with adults. The frequency is lower, but the range of possible causes is wide and early specialist help should be sought if arthritis is suspected.

There are many possible causes of joint problems in children, such as developmental or acquired hip disease, accidents and non-accidental injury. Psychological problems can also declare themselves in children by mimicking joint disorders, with refusal to walk, bizarre gait patterns or complaints of pain. Acute joint infection (septic arthritis – see Chapter 8) is an emergency and if it is suspected the child should be seen by an orthopaedic surgeon or rheumatologist the same day. The joints may become involved in, but not infected by, systemic illnesses such as streptococcal infections or rubella (see also Chapter 8).

The age of a child will make a difference as to how the joint problems declare themselves. Toddlers may just be irritable and reluctant to move, but be unable to express pain in the way that an older child can. A fever is a very important symptom and parents should know how to take their child's temperature.

All children with suspected arthritis should be referred to a paediatrician or paediatric rheumatologist.

Non-infective inflammatory conditions of the joints in childhood

The term juvenile idiopathic arthritis (JIA) is nowadays preferred to older designations such as juvenile rheumatoid arthritis, so as to try to encompass the varieties of inflammatory joint disease in this age group. It is classified into a number of sub-types pragmatically, according to the pattern and type of joint involvement or systemic symptoms. One example is **oligo-articular arthritis**. This means that only a few joints are involved and it has a good outlook as regards the joints. However, there is a risk of eye problems, which have to be monitored carefully. Another type is enthesitis-related, which is like AS in adults.

> **pauci- or oligo-articular arthritis**
> Arthritis affecting a few joints – usually five or fewer.

There is also a juvenile equivalent of adult rheumatoid arthritis, which affects mostly teenagers. Children affected in this way need prolonged specialist treatment to avoid permanent joint damage. Systemic onset juvenile idiopathic arthritis (formerly known as Still's Disease) is a term used to describe children who have a systemic disease, involving the skin, blood and lymph nodes, the arthritis sometimes appearing later on. Systemic lupus erythematosus and vasculitis can also occur in childhood.

Treatment of arthritis in children

The principles are much the same as in adults in terms of medication, with very important differences in terms of dosing and formulation, including the use of liquid preparations. Treatment with steroids has particular implications for a child, in view of its effect on bones that are growing. Physiotherapy, important as it is in adults, is absolutely crucial to the effective treatment of children with arthritis. (The details of the methods are inappropriate for a book like this.) It also should go without saying that the child's educational needs are to be incorporated with the whole programme of management.

CHAPTER

6

Gout and crystal arthritis

What is gout?

The term 'gout' derives from *gutta*, which means 'a drop'. Perhaps the name was adopted because the pain in gout is a little like that experienced when a hot liquid drops onto the foot. Sometimes gout is often assumed to mean any pain in the foot, the most commonly affected part, but this is not so. Gout is due to inflammation produced by crystals of uric acid deposited in joints or soft tissues. Strictly speaking, it is not an acid by the time it forms crystals, but urate. There is another form of arthritis known as 'pseudo-gout', which is due to the accumulation of a different sort of crystal, made from pyrophosphate. It is possible that there are other forms of inflammation due to crystals, producing appearances like gout, which are as yet unidentified.

Symptoms

Acute gout can be extremely painful. If the foot is affected, as it very frequently is, even the pressure of bedclothes becomes unbearable and walking may be impossible until the pain diminishes. The attack often begins at night and accelerates over a few hours. The affected part becomes swollen, red and shiny (see figure 6.1).

The inflammation may be so intense that the skin peels, as it does over a boil or other abscess. Indeed, there are parallels with infection. The inflammatory process is similar and the crystals are handled by the white cells of the body in almost the same way as are bacteria. So it is important that gout is not presumed to be an infection and even more important that an infected joint (i.e. septic arthritis) is not assumed to be gout or any other type of arthritis. This is not necessarily straightforward. It may necessitate a doctor inserting a needle into the joint in question to draw off and test the fluid, which may well be so thick with white cells and crystals that it looks like pus. The microscope photograph of the fluid (see plate 7) shows white cells, debris and thin needle-shaped crystals.

Q Is gout hereditary?

A Yes, quite strongly so in some cases. One might theoretically find a man developing gout in his twenties who is slim, teetotal and a vegetarian, whose father and uncle had gout! Clearly, it would be no great surprise that he might develop it. However, things are much less clear-cut than that.

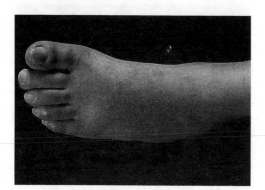

❚ Figure 6.1 Acute gout of the foot.

Q **Is gout getting more common?**

A Possibly so, although not greatly. It is actually the most common form of inflammatory arthritis (more so than rheumatoid arthritis) in middle aged and older men. Around 1 per cent of the UK population are gout sufferers at one time or another.

ketosis
An acid condition of the body which gives a sour smell on the breath.

Patterns of gout

Attacks of acute gout may come out of the blue, or may be precipitated by an acute illness such as pneumonia, by stress such as surgery, or by over-indulgence in a heavy drinking session. These events appear very different but a common theme – dehydration and **ketosis** – links them together. The most familiar example of ketosis is the sour breath after excess alcohol.

Even left untreated, an acute attack of gout will eventually settle, but it may take several weeks to do so. Some people get attacks perhaps only once a year, after a stress as described above. With prompt treatment and resolution of each attack, these people really have very little to worry about in terms of damage to their joints. However, if attacks are frequent they merge into a chronic grumbling arthritis, which may not be anything like as painful as an acute attack, but which may cause persisting joint damage. This is then termed 'chronic gouty arthritis' (see figure 6.2).

It may mimic other forms of arthritis such as rheumatoid arthritis (RA), although it is not

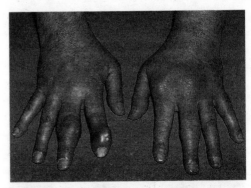

Figure 6.2 The hands of a man with chronic gouty arthritis.

usually as symmetrical in its distribution. (RA tends to involve the joints on both sides of the body to roughly the same degree.) The joints involved become swollen and may be painful, but are still reasonably useable. The patient and even the doctor may be lulled into thinking it will all settle down, but over the months and years the joints may become rather badly damaged (see plate 8).

Q Does gout affect women?

A Women below the age of the menopause rarely develop gout spontaneously. If they do, there is an unusually strong genetic factor, or there may be another cause such as a rare kidney problem. Investigation with this in mind is necessary, or the kidney disease could go unnoticed until it is severe. Older women may develop gout spontaneously, possibly as the influence of oestrogens wane. The most common factor is the increasing numbers of women with heart problems on diuretic drugs.

Soft tissue gout

Gout can affect soft tissues as well as joints. **Tophi** are firm white-ish swellings, often over the ear, or part of the swelling of the hand or foot. They consist of more or less solid urate. This can be proved by removing a tiny sample with a syringe and needle for examination under a microscope. (See figures 6.3–6.5 for examples of this).

Tophi are often painless, but may be removed surgically if they become ulcerated or infected. With prolonged treatment to lower blood urate levels (see below) they may disappear. Urate can accumulate elsewhere, such as in the spine, but this is unusual.

tophi
A collection of uric acid crystals which present as swellings.

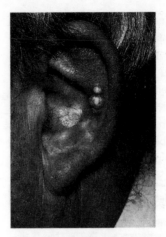

Figure 6.3 Gouty tophus of the ear.

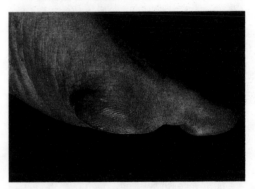

Figure 6.4 Gouty tophus of the foot.

Q Can gout affect children?

A Conventional gout occurs so rarely in children, younger women or adolescent men that it should always be investigated further rather than just accepted as an unusual case of gout. There are some particular causes:

◇ Familial Juvenile Hyperuricaemic Nephropathy — primarily a kidney disorder, which may result in gout

✧ Lesch-Nyhan syndrome and Kelley Seegmiller syndrome — rare inherited enzyme deficiencies
✧ Phosphoribosylpyrophosphate synthetase superactivity (PRPS) syndrome — extremely rare.

Discussion of these is beyond the scope of this book (see further help, page 200).

Uric acid and gout

A raised uric acid level in the blood, termed **hyperuricaemia**, is the single most important risk factor for developing gout. The higher the level, the greater the risk of eventually developing gout and also the higher the risk of developing damage to joints or to the kidney. In one group of men studied for five years, the risk of developing gout was 30 per cent in those with a very high blood level of uric acid and only 0.6 per cent in those with a level that was lower, but still in the hyperuricaemic range.

In addition, the higher the level of uric acid in the blood, the younger a man will be when he gets his first attack and therefore the longer his joints will be exposed to attacks, unless they are prevented.

hyperuricaemia
Raised uric acid (urate) level in the blood.

Q What is the importance of the blood uric acid in gout?

A For practical purposes, gout will not occur in someone who has never had a raised level of uric acid (urate) in the blood.

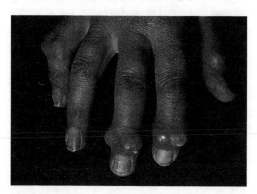

Figure 6.5 Tophi in the hand at osteoarthritic joints.

Q **What should be the level of uric acid in the blood to avoid gout?**

A This is for those familiar with biochemical terms! In men, hyperuricaemia (i.e. a raised blood level of urate) is defined as 0.42 millimoles per litre (=420 micromoles per litre, or 7.0 mgm per 100 mls (or /dL)). In males this adult level is achieved soon after puberty. For adult women before the menopause, the figure is 0.34 millimoles (340 micromoles per litre or 5.7 mgm per 100 mls). After the menopause the level rises somewhat.

Other characteristics that predict the development of hyperuricaemia and therefore of gout include: raised blood pressure (hypertension); the use of water tablets (diuretics); obesity and a high alcohol intake. Diet is discussed below.

Diet

Uric acid circulates in the body as urate, because biochemically it is a weak acid, as distinct from a strong one like hydrochloric acid. It is urate that forms the inflammatory crystals. Uric acid arises from the breakdown of purines; these purines are the result of the natural breakdown of nucleic acids which, in turn, arise from the breakdown of DNA in cell nuclei. A lot of energy goes into making DNA so the human body tries to conserve as much as possible. Therefore, only a limited amount of one's blood uric acid is released from breakdown of one's own cells.

A considerable amount arises from that DNA which is consumed in the diet. If you then consider that the more cells there are in any food, the greater the quantity of DNA, then it is fairly simple to understand which foods are more likely to lead to a high uric acid content. These are the foods that contain lots of nuclei and they are therefore those that are very active, expending energy, making proteins and cell constituents and so forth. A rule of thumb is that anything you eat that has worked hard for its living is likely to contain more cells and therefore more purines. So, for example, the liver and kidneys, which are working all the time whether their owner is asleep or awake, are very dense in nuclei and this offal is particularly prone to lead to high uric acid levels when eaten. Conversely, white meat from chicken breast contains a lower concentration of purines than does the darker meat of chicken legs. Similarly, highly active fish such as sardines, anchovies and salmon, contain more purines than 'couch potato' fish such as plaice. Asparagus, which does grow very fast, is not a particularly important provider of purines because we eat very little of it. Beans, of which we eat more, grow fast and contain a moderate amount of purines. By reducing the amount of offal and red meat in the diet, one is likely to reduce the amount of purine consumed. This will reduce, at least a little, the blood urate level and therefore will lower the likelihood of urate depositing in tissues as crystals.

The level of uric acid may not necessarily need reducing by very much to make a significant difference to the risk of gout: perhaps from just above the upper limit of normal to just within the normal range. This is because the solubility of urate in blood is actually relatively low and it does not take much of a rise above average to get to a level where the urate can come out of solution. The reasons for deposits of urate are complex and not fully understood, and the relationship with blood level is not linear. However, one can say with confidence that for someone to develop gout, his or her blood urate level will have been above average. As was pointed out above, if the level of uric acid remains very high, the likelihood of gout developing is also very high.

If you have gout, or if you are found incidentally to have a raised blood level of uric acid, here are a few pointers to help you with your diet.

Avoid   – liver, kidneys, shellfish, yeast extracts

Reduce – the overall protein intake, especially red meat

Q **Is gout caused by the wrong diet?**

A Not quite. However, diet plays an important role for some people. The apocryphal vegetarian teetotal man with classical gout (incidentally, I have never met one!) may never be able to modify his diet sufficiently to avoid gout, but many others can.

Increase – the vegetable proportion of protein
intake, including soy beans
– fruit intake, especially cherries (fresh
or preserved, including juice)
– skimmed milk and low fat yoghurt
– the proportion of unsaturated fat
from nuts, oils and fish.

Q My doctor says that if I take a drug to lower my uric acid level I need not bother to do anything about my diet, provided I lose a bit of weight.

A Your doctor is partly correct. Some people eat so much meat, offal or shell-fish, or drink so much beer, that dieting to lose weight and to cut down the purine intake might be sufficient to avoid the need for drugs. More often, the dieting enables much easier control and prevention of attacks. In some people, diet plays a minor part (if any at all), in generating excess uric acid, so diet will not make much difference. A diet that is truly low in purine is actually very unpalatable and might be unbalanced in other ways.

Body weight, diabetes and heart problems

Heavier people have higher blood urate levels. This is true, but it is not that simple. The nature of the diet, the sex of the person and the differences in metabolism between people all play a part in dictating the uric acid level; yet other factors influence whether or not gout transpires. Men with gout have a raised risk of cardiovascular disorders such as hypertension (raised blood pressure), stroke and coronary artery disease (heart attacks).

The reasons are complex and not clearly understood, but the associations are sufficiently strong that it is advisable for anyone with gout to have their cholesterol and other blood lipids checked, along with their blood pressure. These factors are related not just to body weight, as measured by BMI (Body Mass Index, which relates body weight to height) but to a certain type of obesity. This 'central' obesity is summarized by having a fat middle. This means men with a waist-to-hip ratio of more than 1.0 and women with a ratio of more than 0.8. Men with a waist measurement of over 90 cm (36 inches) have a higher than average risk of heart and blood vessel disease. This is also linked to Type 2 diabetes, which comes on in adulthood. The underlying problem is summarized as 'insulin resistance'. So it may be that insulin resistance is linked indirectly with a tendency to a raised uric acid level.

> **Point to remember**
> If you develop gout, make sure that you have your blood pressure checked, along with your blood cholesterol and other lipids and a diabetes screen.

Alcohol

Most alcoholic drinks do not contain much in the way of purines, although some beers do. The links between gout and alcohol are several. It is probable that the influence of alcohol is to do with its effects on promoting obesity and, in addition, its tendency to produce higher quantities of weak acids in its metabolism. These are the ketones, such as lactic acid, that produce the sour smell on the breath. These ketones compete with uric acid for excretion by the kidney and thereby cause the blood uric acid to rise.

myth
Gout only occurs in wealthy men who drink port.

fact
That may have been partly true in days gone by, when most people worked physically hard or could not afford to eat enough to get fat. Port was popular among the better off, but this stereotype may never have been truly accurate and is certainly not the case nowadays. Beer is more likely to lead to gout than spirits or even wine.

Other drinks

Anyone with gout should avoid dehydration, even if there is no history of kidney stones. In fact it is probably sensible to drink plenty of water: several pints a day in one form or another. Tea or coffee is best restricted to three to four cups a day, because more might dehydrate; they also contain methylxanthines such as caffeine and theo-bromine, which theoretically could contribute to purine levels if they or other caffeinated drinks are consumed to excess. Hence you should stick mostly to water or a variety of fruit juices.

People with a history of kidney stones will especially be advised to drink two to three litres of water a day. They may need to try to increase the pH of their urine (to make the urine more alkaline than usual) by taking sodium citrate or bicarbonate which unfortunately are not very palatable.

Gout and the kidney

In the early half of the twentieth century, chronic kidney (renal) disease was seen in up to 40 per cent of patients with gout. Renal failure was the cause of death in 25 per cent. Stones in the kidney or bladder can occur in patients with gout who excrete larger than average amounts of uric acid in their urine. There is a particular tendency for some to do this, perhaps because of a genetically linked variation in the way that their kidneys operate. These 'stone formers' make up about 1 per cent of patients with gout.

Progressive kidney failure in patients with gout is now unusual. It is mainly limited to inadequately treated patients with rare forms of inherited kidney disease, chronic lead poisoning or other kidney disease.

People who have had a kidney transplant are prone to develop gout: they are likely to be advised about this as part of their medical care. People who have had a heart transplant are even more liable to develop gout, probably because of the medicines required to suppress rejection.

Treatment

Herbal remedies

Many natural or herbal remedies are marketed for gout. These include celery seeds, garlic, artichoke, saponins and combinations of these and others. Cherries have already been mentioned and remain the only food constituent remedy for which there is some scientific evidence. However, as has been said before, the lack of evidence *for* benefit is not necessarily evidence of *lack* of effect. So, provided the risks of not treating gout are accepted, there is no reason why a person with definite gout should not try such remedies first, before resorting to medication.

Medication

There are two aspects: the treatment of the acute attack and the prevention of future attacks.

The acute attack is often extremely painful, especially if it is the first ever. The intense inflammatory pain can be eased a bit by applying an ice pack, if its weight can be tolerated. Always put a tea-towel or something similar between the ice (or frozen peas) and the skin, or an 'ice burn' can occur. The affected joint, which is the foot in over half of all cases, is usually too painful to use so the patient needs no advice to rest!

In terms of drug treatment, the following are effective:

✧ non-steroidal anti-inflammatory drugs (NSAIDs). Examples include diclofenac and naproxen
✧ colchicine
✧ a course of steroid tablets (prednisolone) or a steroid injection, into the muscle for absorption into the system, or into the joint if feasible.

Each of these drugs has its own potential side-effect problems, but mostly these can be overcome. The dosage is a matter for the prescribing doctor, taking into account the patient's medical history.

NSAIDs

If the NSAID approach is taken, the dose needed to suppress an attack of gout should probably be rather greater than the normal maintenance dosage. Purely as an example, the normal maintenance dose of naproxen is 500–1000 mgm per day, given as two doses, each of 250 or 500 mgm tablets. For acute gout, the dose may need to be increased to 1500 mgm per day for three to four days, thereafter reverting down to the usual dose. On this regimen, most attacks will settle within ten days, often much less. Once the diagnosis is made, the sooner the treatment starts, the better. Once a gout patient has had one attack, they can usually diagnose themselves from then on.

Some people cannot tolerate NSAIDs because of nausea or abdominal pain, nor should they try to persevere. Another medicine may be prescribed alongside the NSAID to offset these stomach problems. Examples include cimetidine or omeprazole, both of which reduce stomach acid secretion. In principle one prefers not to give one drug to offset the side-effects of another, but sometimes beggars cannot be choosers.

Using colchicine

If NSAIDs cannot be tolerated, then the colchicine approach can be considered. Indeed, some doctors would recommend colchicine as the first line of treatment over an NSAID.

This drug (pronounced kol-che-seen) is derived from the crocus. Like many drugs still in use, it has a longstanding herbal background. Its mode of action is quite different from an NSAID and it is not effective in any of the other common forms of arthritis, such as osteoarthritis. The predominant side-effects are on the gastrointestinal tract, with nausea, vomiting and/or diarrhoea. Some patients are especially prone to these, in which case they will not be able to tolerate an effective dose. To start with, the dose of one tablet of 0.5 mgm (500 micrograms) is taken about every three hours to a maximum of around 5 mgm before reducing the frequency to maintenance levels of one to two tablets per day. Incidentally, a common US preparation of colchicine is 0.6 mgm. Once the pain starts to ease up, the dosage can be reduced. There is a preparation of colchicine for intravenous injection, but this is best avoided.

Using steroids

Some people, especially if elderly or with heart or kidney problems, have to avoid both NSAIDs and colchicine because of the risk of side-effects. For these, steroid drugs such as prednisolone are actually safer in the short term. Usual dosages for an acute attack would be 15–30 mgm for a week or so; alternatively, a single intra-muscular injection of, for example, methylprednsisolone 40–60 mgm may be very effective and well tolerated.

Prevention of gout

Having paid close attention to diet and lifestyle as discussed above, sooner or later the question of drug treatment will crop up.

Q I get about one attack of gout each year. I can control it within a day or two by taking the anti-inflammatory medicines or colchicine prescribed by my doctor. Am I risking damage to my health by not taking medication to prevent attacks?

A Quite possibly not. There is no absolute answer to this. Provided the attacks are indeed rapidly controlled and provided you know that your general health is good (weight, exercise tolerance, blood pressure etc.) you are taking little risk. If you already have osteoarthritis, this may possibly be accelerated by gouty attacks, although the evidence for this is scanty. Frequent attacks of gout, with consequent prolonged exposure of the joints to inflammation, are likely to lead to joint damage. If this is the case, you should really try to prevent attacks.

The first way of preventing attacks is to take colchicine or a NSAID prophylactically (preventively). This might be effective in preventing (or rather, suppressing) attacks. However, if it is necessary to do this on a daily basis, it almost certainly means that there is chronic grumbling inflammation in the joints. Also, if the blood level of uric acid remains high enough to cause continuous attacks, there might be a risk of kidney damage or stone formation. Finally, the risk of side-effects from continuous NSAID is appreciable. The risks of long-term colchicine are less well documented. Overall, therefore, this is not the best approach.

There are two main medication methods of reducing blood urate levels and therefore reducing the risk of gouty attacks. The first method involves interfering with metabolism in order to reduce the production of uric acid in the body (uricostatic drugs). Until recently, there was only one in general use: allopurinol. For 30 years this has been the most effective way of preventing gout. It inhibits the enzyme xanthine oxidase, which is critical to the process of breaking down purines to uric acid. The pathway is diverted to other substances that are more soluble than urate.

The level of urate in the blood falls within a week or two of starting the drug, which is best introduced with a gradual increase in dose. It is, however, many months before the liability to acute attacks is reduced. Colchicine or an NSAID has to be taken along with the allopurinol for at least several months and maybe a year or so, before a gouty person may be confident enough to continue on allopurinol alone. Even then he or she might need acute treatment from time to time.

Allopurinol is not all wonderful: some patients have nasty hypersensitive reactions with a rash or other problems. For them, the alternatives are to try de-sensitization (a complex business, involving tiny doses of allopurinol and then gradually increasing them) or to try a related drug, called oxipurinol, which is available on a restricted licence on a named-patient basis. Otherwise, treatment usually has to be changed to a uricosuric drug – see below.

Recently febuxostat, a new drug unrelated to allopurinol has been licensed. It is too early at the time of writing to be able to appraise it thoroughly, but the signs are encouraging.

The second method is by causing an increase in the excretion of uric acid by the kidney into the urine with a **uricosuric** drug. Because of the success of allopurinol, uricosurics are used very little in the UK. There is, however, more choice, with three drugs currently available: Sulfinpyrazone, Probenecid and Benzbromarone.

Probenecid and Sulfinpyrazone have been available for many years, but have been supplanted almost entirely by allopurinol. Both may give rise to problems such as nausea, rash or other side-effects. The same precautions as for allopurinol are necessary during the introductory period.

Benzbromarone has been much more widely used in the rest of Europe than in the UK. It is more potent than either Probenecid or Sulfinpyrazone and it probably should be considered more frequently in the UK. Unlike these two, it is effective at reducing urate levels in people with poor kidney function. However, like these two, it is to be avoided in people with a history of any sort of kidney stones, especially urate stones, as it increases still further the amount of urate in the urine. More of a problem is that it has no general licence in the UK, so it has to be specially ordered. There have been reports of liver side-effects, so monitoring is necessary.

uricosuric
A drug which causes excretion of uric acid.

Other drugs for treating gout

The lipid-lowering drug Fenofibrate has some effect in lowering urate. This might be useful if a patient with gout also has a need to reduce blood lipid levels. The blood pressure treatment drug Losartan also reduces blood urate levels. Since patients with gout often do need blood pressure control, this is another possible approach.

Uricase

In rare instances a patient may have such a high level of uric acid, for example, when being treated for certain forms of cancer, that it is important to dissolve the accumulated deposits and allopurinol may not work fast enough. In these rare instances, there are preparations of the enzyme **uricase** available. This is an enzyme that has been lost by humans in the evolutionary process but which is retained by most mammals, which therefore do not suffer from gout. There is no place for this drug, which is given intravenously, in the normal management of gout, because of problems with hypersensitivity and of cost.

uricase
An enzyme that breaks down uric acid to form a more soluble compound, called allantoin. Uricase is present in most animal species but humans have lost it through evolution, so they can get gout!

Steroids

There is almost no place for long-term steroids in the prevention of gout.

Drugs that should be avoided

The principal group of drugs to be avoided is the diuretic drugs, which are used to make people with heart disease excrete more fluid and also to treat hypertension. Any of the diuretics are liable to cause retention of urate and ultimately gout.

This probably explains the increased numbers of older women with gout, as the frequency of heart disease and blood pressure problems in older people, taken with the longer life of females, means that there are probably more women than men on diuretics. The characteristics of diuretic-induced gout are a little different from spontaneous primary gout. The attacks are often at other sites such as the hands. They may not be as acute and may go undiagnosed. Diuretic-induced gout may also coincide with, and be confused with, OA.

Another drug that can cause gout is pyrazinamide, used in the treatment of TB (tuberculosis). This is well known and should be anticipated in that instance.

Pseudo gout

This is discussed in Chapter 2, page 10.

> **Q** My uncle had gout. I have never had an attack and I am 55. Our occupational nurse checked my uric acid as part of a health screen. It was found to be slightly increased. Should I take allopurinol, like my uncle, to prevent gout damaging my joints?

> **A** Your uric acid may have been raised for years. The higher the level, the more likely is gout, but at only slightly above the normal range, the risk of gout is still low. The principle 'prevention is better than cure' should not be applied universally. Your risk of developing gout may still be quite low. It takes many attacks to damage joints. Provided other aspects of your health are satisfactory, such as your blood pressure, then you are better off not taking medication for something that might never happen.

CHAPTER

7

Systemic rheumatic diseases

The description of systemic rheumatic diseases is quite generalized and includes the following diagnoses:

✧ **systemic lupus erythematosus (SLE)** and closely related conditions
✧ scleroderma and systemic sclerosis
✧ inflammatory muscle disease (includes polymyositis and dermatomyositis)
✧ Sjögren's syndrome (primary and secondary types)
✧ systemic vasculitis (includes Wegener's syndrome, Churg-Strauss syndrome and polyarteritis).

People who develop a systemic rheumatic disease may not necessarily develop arthritis with progressive joint damage, although joint pain, swelling, stiffness and even deformity is typically experienced at one time or another. Overall, the possibility of severe illness is higher with this group of conditions, so most patients will be referred to a hospital department for care.

> **systemic lupus erythematosus (SLE)**
> A condition which can give rise to a wide range of symptoms, including arthritis, fevers, skin rashes and kidney problems.

Systemic lupus erythematosus (SLE) and related conditions

'Erythema' means redness and the word 'erythematosus' refers to the red facial rash that often affects patients. The 'lupus' bit may be explained by the resemblance to 'lupus vulgaris', an old name for tuberculosis infections of the face, or by the shape of the facial rash resembling a wolf's face or mask.

> **Q What is lupus?**
>
> **A** It is a systemic rheumatic disease or disorder. In fact it is really a multi-system disorder, because that implies not only is it localized to no single tissue (e.g. the outer layer of the skin) or organ (e.g. the liver), but typically affects more than one system (e.g. the joints, the skin and the lungs). It is characterized by inflammation, but of a rather different sort from that seen in rheumatoid arthritis or ankylosing spondylitis (see question on complement and inflammation in lupus opposite).

The causes of lupus

The genetic background of a patient is important. Although lupus can run quite strongly in families (e.g. in both twins, or a mother and daughter), more often there is a tendency for relatives of patients with lupus to have autoimmune diseases. Thyroid disease is the most common, but others may include rheumatoid arthritis (RA), thrombocytopenic purpura, myasthenia gravis or Type 1 (juvenile onset) diabetes mellitus. This tendency to autoimmune problems is therefore manifesting itself in different ways, perhaps because of variations in genetics or in an environmental trigger. Infections are obvious candidates, but no single infective agent, whether bacteria or virus, has been identified, so there probably isn't one single culprit. The linking theme here is that many patients with lupus have an inherited deficiency in, or disorder of, the complement system. Sunlight (ultraviolet light) is another potent environmental trigger for some patients.

Q I have read about something called 'complement and lupus'. What is complement and why is it relevant to inflammation in lupus?

A Complement is a body defence system against infection that is very ancient in biological evolutionary terms. It is a set of proteins that can stick to bacteria, viruses or fungi and resist their spread or destroy them, with the help of white cells and antibodies. The combination of complement with **antigen** (a bit of a bacterial wall, for example) and an **antibody** is called an immune complex. Patients with lupus probably develop the condition because they are not very good at coping with particular immune complexes. Instead of being cleared away by the lymphatic system and spleen, the complexes continue to circulate widely in the blood and accumulate in places like the kidney where they cause inflammation. This immune complex inflammation may involve elements of the clotting system and tends to be much less full of white cells compared to the synovitis of RA or the enthesitis of the spondylarthropathies.

antigen
A protein that sticks to an antibody forming an immune complex.

antibody
An immunoglobulin protein that sticks to an antigen, such as a bacterium.

Making the diagnosis

The diagnosis is derived from symptoms and clinical findings, with the help of characteristic blood test results. A biopsy (removing a very small piece of tissue, for example, from the skin, for examination under a microscope) is quite often necessary for diagnosing skin rashes or kidney problems. The list below shows the details that were identified by the American College of Rheumatology as being so characteristic that the presence of four or more of them are suggestive of the diagnosis. However, these criteria are *not designed for diagnosis*. They are to make sure that when doctors are comparing groups of people diagnosed as SLE, they are using the same concepts.

For example, a patient may have arthritis; she may have had mouth ulcers in the past; she may have had an attack of pleurisy and she may have kidney disease. She still might not have SLE, as each of these features may have another explanation. So it is implicit in this list that the features must have no other explanation, for them to be taken as evidence of SLE. On the other hand a patient may develop, say, photosensitivity in 2003 then, in 2005, arthritis. Shortly afterwards she might note a facial rash and a blood test reveals an abnormally low white cell count. She now has SLE: but clearly she has probably really had it since 2003. So the criteria necessary to allocate the patient to the SLE group for comparison purposes do not have to be simultaneously present.

The American College of Rheumatology criteria for SLE

1 Characteristic rash across the cheek.
2 Discoid lesion rash.
3 Photosensitivity.
4 Oral ulcers.
5 Arthritis.
6 Inflammation of membranes in the lungs, the heart, or the abdomen.
7 Evidence of kidney disease.

8 Evidence of severe neurological disease.
9 Haematological (blood) disorders, such as low red or white blood cell and platelet counts.
10 Immunological abnormalities.
11 Positive antinuclear antibody (ANA).

The symptoms of lupus (SLE)

Lupus has a very wide variety of possible manifestations. Below is a list of the more common features. Of course, they are not present simultaneously or indeed necessarily at any time. Virtually none is unique to lupus, although some are characteristic.

Common manifestations of lupus

The most common features of lupus include:

✧ general symptoms of fatigue, fever and weight loss
✧ arthritis
✧ skin rashes
✧ kidney disease
✧ lung and heart disease
✧ blood disorders (low white count, anaemia)
✧ neurological disorders.

General symptoms

Fatigue is extremely common, as is aching in muscles and joints. Therefore, if someone is tired and run-down but is also one of those people who has a positive **anti-nuclear antibody** (ANA) by chance (as some do), there is a risk of an inappropriate diagnosis of lupus. Other generalized symptoms that are common in lupus include weight loss and low-grade fever (less than about 38° C or 100° F).

Q Who gets lupus?

A If you develop lupus below the age of 50, you are 90 per cent likely to be a woman (and of course very likely to be pre-menopausal). If over 50, the ratio evens up somewhat. Children can, rarely, develop it. It is much more common in black, Asian and Chinese people than in Europeans. The relevance of inheritance has been mentioned. There are definite environmental factors in some patients. Best known are ultraviolet light and some pharmaceutical medicines.

anti-nuclear antibody
An autoantibody positive in 95–8 per cent of patients with lupus.

Joints

Most patients with lupus get joint pain (arthralgia) at one time or another. It varies from day to day and pain is often more prominent than in other types of arthritis. Some patients become so affected by weariness, pain and aching all over that they have actually reacted in a fibromyalgia type of way. So it is not really surprising that fibromyalgia is sometimes regarded as an autoimmune condition. There can be distortion of the fingers or toes which is due to contractures (shortening) of the tendons more than to erosion of the bone and cartilage of the joints, as in RA (see figure 7.1). A particular form of joint damage called **avascular necrosis** is relatively more common in lupus. It results in severe damage to the end of a bone (such as the hip) and occurs in very active disease which results in the necessity to give treatment with high doses of steroids.

avascular necrosis
The impairment of blood supply to a bone, usually within a joint, causing it to collapse. Can occur spontaneously or can be caused by very high doses of corticosteroids.

Skin

Lupus causes many different types of rash. The most well known is a butterfly rash on the face and, although characteristic of lupus, this does

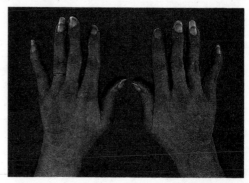

Figure 7.1 Hands of a patient with lupus arthritis.

not mean that everyone develops it (see plate 9). It presents as a red rash over the cheeks, the nose and chin – the 'blush' area of the face. It looks like sunburn, and in some ways it is. An exaggerated tendency to react to ultraviolet light, with sunburn (photosensitivity) is experienced by about half of all patients. Other rashes include **urticaria**, **discoid lupus** (localized patches of inflammation) and **lupus profundus** (deeper skin lesions).

> **urticaria**
> An itchy rash.

> **discoid lupus and lupus profundus**
> Particular types of rash associated with lupus.

A dermatologist is often needed to decide if a rash is, or is not, due to lupus. In fact, many lupus experts are dermatologists and combined clinics are often held between rheumatologists and dermatologists because of the frequency of skin problems. A specialist assessment of the type of ultraviolet light to which a patient may be sensitive is sometimes required, to identify the appropriate protection required. An increase in hair loss is quite common, especially when the disease is active. Bald patches may appear but fortunately overall baldness (alopecia) is rare. Mouth ulcers are another feature of active disease. **Purpura** means a type of bruise due to multiple little bleeds into the skin, often due to an abnormally low platelet count. An excessive tendency to bruising may also be due to steroids or to aspirin.

> **purpura**
> A purplish rash due to little patches of bleeding into the skin.

Livedo reticularis is a reddish-purple network appearance, usually over the extremities (see figure 7.2). It has several causes other than lupus, but is especially frequent in people with lupus who have the anti-phospholipid antibodies (see page 129). It is evidence of stasis (slowing or stopping) of the blood flow through small skin blood vessels and is more obvious in the cold.

> **livedo reticularis**
> A reddish-purple rash usually found over the extremities.

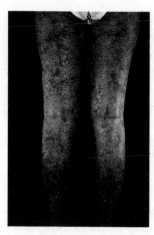

❚ Figure 7.2 Livedo reticularis rash.

Circulatory problems

Raynaud's phenomenon is a reversible alteration in the circulation to the fingers which can also sometimes present elsewhere (see plate 10). Although it may occur in SLE, it is most frequent in scleroderma (see page 140). It varies considerably in severity: first there is a phase when the fingers go white (**ischaemia**), then blueish-purple (stasis phase), then they flush red and tingle. Vasculitis means blood vessel inflammation and may show itself as a patchy, itchy discoloration around the fingertips or elsewhere. It also varies greatly in severity and may occur in any of the systemic rheumatic conditions. Being prone to chilblains does not mean that you necessarily have lupus, but they are quite common, and may be severe enough to require steroid or hydroxychloroquine treatment.

Raynaud's phenomenon
A reversible spasm of blood vessels – normally in the fingers.

ischaemia
A shortage of blood supply.

Chest and heart

Possible lung problems in lupus include pleurisy, pleural effusions, and **pneumonitis**. Quite a

pneumonitis
Inflammation of the lungs.

common symptom is pain down the centre of the chest, with no abnormality to be found either on examination or X-ray. The heart is occasionally affected by inflammation (pericarditis) in a way similar to pleurisy; rarely, the valves can become inflamed and damaged.

Late-onset cardiovascular disease in lupus

The frequency of heart attacks (coronary thrombosis or myocardial infarction), hypertension (raised blood pressure), stroke and poor circulation in the legs is increased in patients who have had lupus for some years. This is probably due partly to the general impact of prolonged inflammation on the body and partly to steroid treatment. It means that doctors and patients have to be alert to all ways of reducing the risks of developing these complications.

Kidney disorder

Inflammation of the kidney (**nephritis**) is one of the more common severe types of lupus. It is associated with the presence of anti-DNA antibodies, which may actually cause it. It can usually be detected early on provided the urine is tested regularly for blood, protein and also for casts, which are microscopic evidence of cells and protein. It causes raised blood pressure, reduced excretion of waste products, such as urea, and sometimes water retention with **oedema** (swelling of the legs). In very severe cases the kidneys may fail to work properly: the condition of renal failure. In these exceptional cases, renal dialysis or transplantation can be successful.

nephritis
Inflammation of the kidney.

oedema
Accumulation of fluid in the legs.

Gastrointestinal problems

This includes the liver, the stomach and the rest of the intestinal tract (the small and the large bowel). Diarrhoea sometimes occurs in active lupus for no very obvious reason. Inflammation of the liver (hepatitis) can sometimes occur, but the most common problem is probably disturbance of liver function as shown by raised liver enzymes in the blood (usually the ALT, AST or Gamma GT), so these tests are standard screening tests for lupus patients. These abnormalities may also be caused by medication.

Lymphopoietic system

This includes the lymph nodes (such as the glands around the neck, under the armpit or in the groin), the spleen (under the ribs on the left side of the abdomen), the liver (under the ribs on the right side of the abdomen) and the bone marrow. Lymphadenopathy (enlargement of the lymph glands) often occurs early as part of the general over-activity of the immune system. Sometimes it precedes clinical symptoms and lead to surgical removal of a gland for diagnostic purposes. Enlargement of the spleen (spleno-megaly) or the liver (hepatomegaly) usually means that there is abnormal function, such as haemolytic anaemia, when the red cells are destroyed faster than normal in the spleen.

The nervous system

Either or both the central (the brain) or the peripheral nervous system (the nerves) can be affected by inflammation. This is a worrying development for everyone, but it may be limited to headaches or migraines that can be controlled with medication. More severe involvement, such as mood disturbance, confusion or epilepsy will need careful assessment and treatment.

Subtypes or associated types of lupus

The anti-phospholipid syndrome

This can exist by itself or as part of lupus. Phospholipids are chemical groups present on lots of different cell membranes. Antibodies to them (probably actually to protein groups linked with the lipids) therefore range widely in their consequences. These possibilities include:

✧ recurrent thrombosis in arteries or veins anywhere in the body
✧ livedo reticularis, which is a characteristic skin appearance (see page 125)
✧ recurrent miscarriages
✧ migraines
✧ a low platelet count (thrombocytopenia) causing bleeding.

Aspirin is probably sufficient for those who have not actually had a thrombosis. Effective anti-coagulation with the drugs warfarin or heparin is essential for some. The place of warfarin as a prophylactic (preventive) treatment in patients who have anti-phospholipid antibodies but have not had a thrombosis is not yet certain.

Drug-induced lupus

The symptoms of this are similar to spontaneous SLE, apart from kidney disease, which does not seem to occur. Skin rashes and fever are relatively common. Between 30 and 40 different drugs have been claimed to cause cases of lupus, but the risks of it happening are very low for any of these apart from three (procainamide, quinidine and hydrallazine) that are anyway seldom used nowadays. However, whenever the question of lupus arises, because of symptoms or because of abnormal blood tests such as the ANA, any current medication should be taken into account.

The management of lupus

People with lupus *may* become very ill and die. It is always *potentially* a dangerous condition and should be taken seriously. A short review in a book like this cannot be interpreted to make predictions for the individual patient.

Having sounded alarm bells, it is also important to point out (again!) that the diagnosis is sometimes made inappropriately, on the grounds of a positive blood test. The range of lupus symptoms is very wide; it can fade away completely; and it can reasonably often be controlled with treatment.

The outlook for active, symptomatic lupus is best where the patient attends a specialized service, rather than seeing a doctor who has limited experience of the condition. In the 1940s few patients would survive five years from diagnosis, whereas nowadays over 90 per cent do. That is not to be complacent: lupus can still be fatal and the survival rate of 95 per cent at five years but only 85 per cent at ten years is not too reassuring for a 25-year-old. There is such a wide range of possible ways for the condition to evolve, including clearing up completely, that it can be misleading to generalize. Nephritis can cause renal failure but treatment can suppress the inflammation satisfactorily. Low white counts can be worrying, but may stabilize and cause no harm. Avascular necrosis may require joint

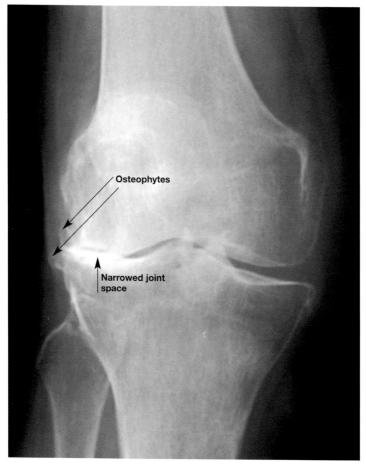

Plate 1 A knee joint in osteoarthritis.

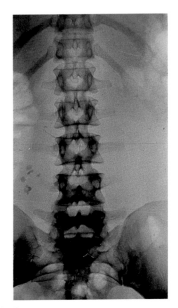

Plate 2(a) A normal spine.

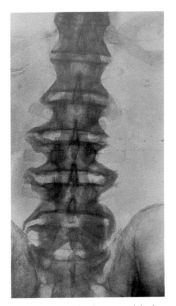

Plate 2(b) A spine showing advanced lumbar spondylosis.

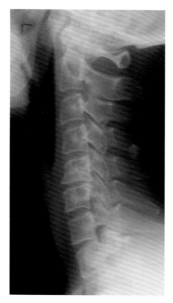

Plate 3 An X-ray of the neck showing an abnormally straight spine.

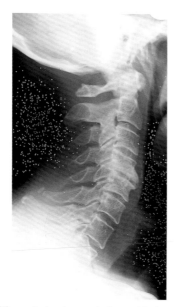

Plate 4 An X-ray of the neck showing cervical spondylosis.

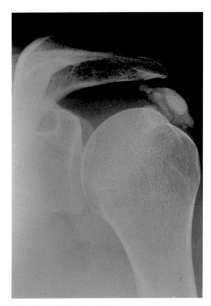

Plate 5   An X-ray showing calcific bursitis.

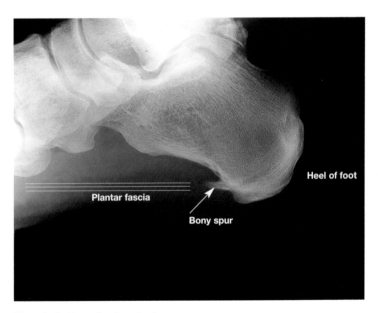

Heel of foot

Plantar fascia

Bony spur

Plate 6   An X-ray showing a heel spur.

This is a white blood cell. The resolution of the picture does not give much detail, but the cell is most likely to be a polymorphonuclear leucocyte.

This shows a crystal inside a cell. Leucocytes engulf crystals, releasing the inflammatory proteins which cause the pain and swelling of gout.

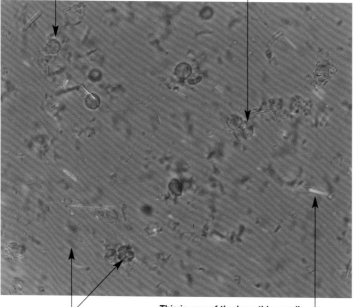

There is also a certain amount of debris, for example from bits of cells that have died.

This is one of the long thin needle-shaped crystals of urate (uric acid) that are characteristic of gout.

Plate 7 A specimen of synovial fluid from the joint of a patient with gout.

These 'empty spaces' are cysts in the lower end of the tibia bone at the ankle. A space like this is particularly characteristic of chronic gouty arthritis. The bone has been slowly replaced at this point by inflammatory tissue which does not show up on the X-ray, so it looks like an empty space.

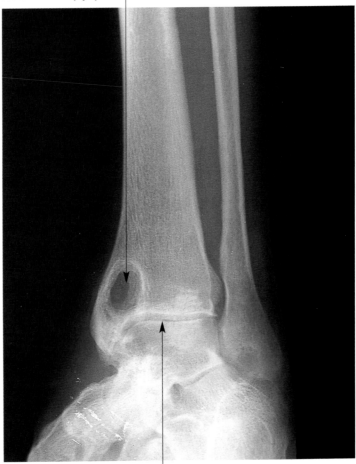

Here the joint space between the ends of the bones is just starting to be reduced. Gout tends not to damage the cartilage as early as, for example, rheumatoid arthritis, but it will do so after a few years of repeated attacks of gout.

Plate 8 An X-ray showing an ankle with gouty damage to the bones.

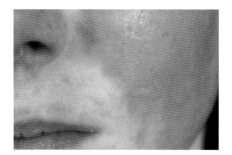

Plate 9 Butterfly rash.

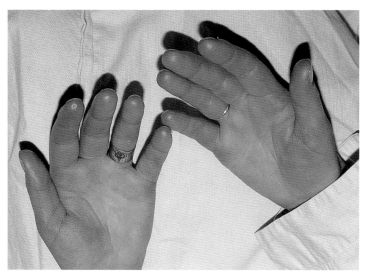

Plate 10 Raynaud's phenomenon.

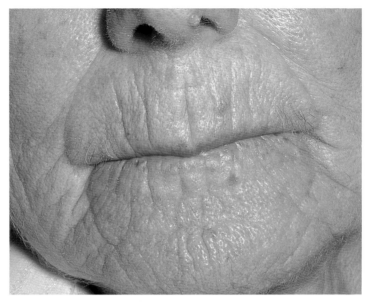

Plate 11 A mouth with telangiectasia in scleroderma.

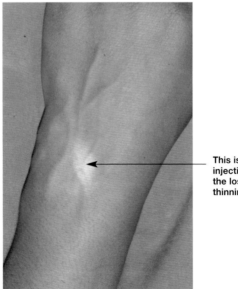

This is the site of the injection of steroid, showing the loss of pigment and thinning of the skin.

Plate 12 This person had a cortico-steroid injection into the wrist to relieve inflammatory arthritis. Steroid injections do not always result in this effect and pigmented skin reveals it more clearly. The change will diminish with time, but it does remind one that steroid injection may have marked effects.

replacement, but the outlook for such surgery is mostly satisfactory.

The following is a summary of how medical treatment can be regarded.

Lifestyle management

Fear of the unknown promotes anxiety, sleeplessness and fatigue. Patients should seek to know as much about their own situation as possible, rather than presuming the worst. Therefore, education is a crucial aspect of treating patients with lupus. If family and friends also understand the situation, it is easier to cope with the 'ups and downs' of lupus. A patient may need to sleep for longer than usual during a flare: yet exercise is important, once the flare has settled, to regain physical fitness. If patients make themselves aware of the possible problems associated with medication, they feel more comfortable with their treatment. If they are familiar with the roles of the medical and nursing teams treating them, they will know when they can consult their doctor for advice and when to ring for an earlier hospital appointment.

Since many lupus patients are working when they develop the condition, the question of their individual ability and willingness to continue to work may require discussion with family, partner and employer. Life and sickness insurance raises difficult issues. Again, information is the key: an insurer may take a more lenient view if they have more information than just the label: 'Has systemic lupus erythematosus'.

The growing awareness of long-term cardio-vascular damage in lupus has been mentioned already. A diet aimed at ideal weight and minimizing cardiovascular risk is an important

Q **Can lupus be cured? Or does it ever burn itself out?**

A No, lupus is never cured in the sense that antibiotics can cure an infection. However, some young women patients can have really quite severe lupus, involving perhaps the kidneys or the blood, which needs powerful treatment to be controlled, but then it seems to go into remission: what amounts to an 'attack' of lupus that does seem to burn itself out.

adjunct to medication. There is no such thing as a special diet for lupus. Salt, fat and refined sugars should be reduced to below what many people eat and a high intake of fibre is encouraged. Extra vitamins are unnecessary when fresh fruit and vegetables are taken daily, as they should be.

Contraception

The female preponderance means that most patients with lupus below the age of 50 are either mothers with children at home or are women considering future motherhood. Overall, fertility is about average, but patients with the anti-phospholipid syndrome (see page 129) may have repeated miscarriages. There is a theoretical risk that female hormones (oestrogens) could cause flares, but it appears that in practice, with modern contraceptive pills, this is not usually a problem. If there is concern about oestrogen-induced flare or thrombosis, and if condoms or cap methods are not regarded as sufficiently secure, the progestogen-only pill or injection can be prescribed. It is a good idea for women to discuss their individual situation with a doctor or family planning clinic.

Planning a family

This is a very personal issue and lupus adds another consideration: should you defer pregnancy until everything is under control or go ahead and have a family as soon as possible? Women are more likely to feel like embarking on pregnancy during a good phase of their illness. However, it might be considered better to go ahead with a pregnancy anyhow, because it might be better to be young with lupus and a baby, than older with lupus and a baby! Matters such as maternity leave,

Q Can drugs used for lupus affect fertility?

A Cyclophosphamide, in particular, can do so. Prolonged treatment (that is, many months or years) with cyclophosphamide may suppress ovarian function, resulting in infertility and early menopause. NSAIDs can reduce fertility, but this is very unusual.

work commitments, support networks and childcare should all be taken into account.

The effect of lupus on pregnancy

Kidney disease (nephritis) requires especially careful observation during pregnancy, to monitor blood pressure and kidney function. A normal vaginal delivery is often possible, but early induction may be required. It is sometimes difficult to tell the difference between a lupus flare and **pre-eclampsia**, as both may involve a raised blood pressure and increased protein in the urine.

The effect of lupus on the baby

If the mother's lupus is well controlled and factors such as blood pressure are normal, the baby is likely to be healthy. However, there are two particular aspects requiring elaboration: maternal antibodies (anti-Ro antibodies – see below) and medication.

> **pre-eclampsia**
> A disorder that can occur during pregnancy. It includes raised blood pressure and protein in the urine. It can be dangerous for mother and baby and needs urgent attention and treatment.

> **Anti-Ro antibodies**
> It is normal for antibodies in a healthy woman to pass across the placenta into the baby's circulation, thereby providing protection to the baby until its immune system has matured. Some women with lupus have antibodies called anti-Ro in their blood; in a small proportion (about one twentieth) of these, conduction problems in the baby's heart can result. Since this is a specific problem linked with anti-Ro, it can be anticipated and usually managed safely. There is a syndrome called neonatal lupus, in which different antibodies may play a part, but this is extremely unusual. Other antibodies found in lupus patients, such as anti-nuclear antibodies, very rarely provide a risk for the baby.

Medication during pregnancy

The medication list should be carefully scrutinized before embarking on pregnancy in order to withdraw any that might be troublesome to the baby. Drugs that suppress the immune system, such as cyclophosphamide, are usually avoided completely. Others, such as hydroxychloroquine, are probably safe, but most mothers and doctors prefer to err on the safe side. Anti-inflammatory drugs can, very rarely, reduce fertility or can cause problems during the final stages of pregnancy as the woman goes into labour, so are withdrawn at that stage. Steroids may have to be increased to compensate for the withdrawal of, for example, azathioprine, and this increase can cause problems in the baby. These are usually temporary. Pregnant women with lupus should not be tempted to take complementary medicines without consulting their doctors.

myth
Women with lupus should not risk getting pregnant.

fact
It is true that lupus may provide additional risks to both mother and baby. However, they can usually be managed safely, provided that there is close supervision during pregnancy.

Treatment

(See also Chapter 10 for further details of the individual drugs.)

This can be divided for discussion into the treatment of symptoms and particular problems and treatment aimed at suppressing the disease.

Symptom- and problem-related treatment

This covers treating symptoms such as pain and also problems that arise during the course of lupus, such as infection, depression or raised blood pressure. Examples include:

✧ pain – requiring medication such as paracetamol, codeine or anti-inflammatory drugs such as ibuprofen

✧ infection – a very important aspect, as fever can be due to active lupus or to infection complicating it, so diagnosis must be accurate and antibiotic treatment precisely tailored to the bacterium responsible

✧ thrombosis – managed with medication such as aspirin, warfarin or heparin

✧ poor circulation, such as Raynaud's or vasculitis – managed with drugs that dilate blood vessels (vasodilators), such as nifedipine or prostacycline

✧ epilepsy – treated with anti-convulsant drugs.

Disease-suppressing treatment

Most of the problems attributable directly to lupus are concerned in some way with inflammation. As outlined above, it is somewhat different from the joint inflammation in RA, so although some of the approaches are similar, there are important differences.

Non-steroidal anti-inflammatory drugs (NSAIDs) are often useful, for example, to control arthralgia (painful joints), chest pain due to pleurisy or perhaps to facilitate a lower dose of steroids. Hydroxychloroquine, which is most well known as an anti-malarial drug, is quite effective in controlling lupus skin inflammation. It is also helpful for arthralgia and pleuritic pains. The maximum dose for prolonged treatment is 400 mgm a day and it takes between three and six weeks to start working. Chloroquine is an older, related, drug but is rarely used now, because it has to be regularly monitored to detect early eye damage. Dapsone and Mepacrine are also used for a wide range of conditions including malaria and leprosy but can be helpful, with careful monitoring, for lupus rashes.

Steroids are really the mainstay of treatment: almost all patients with lupus will have to take this drug in some form at one time or another. The usual form in the UK is prednisolone. Prednisone is the form preferred in the USA but for most people there is no difference: prednisone is broken down in the liver to form prednisolone, which is the active drug. The dose required to suppress symptoms and improve function may have to be as high as 1 mgm for each kilogramme of body weight, but the usual practice will be to take between 5 and 20 mgm each day, increasing to 30 to 40 mgm to control a flare-up.

Q I know steroids can be very dangerous: how can I reduce their side-effects?

A The list of possible steroid side-effects is quite long. It includes raised blood pressure, excessive weight gain, bruising, osteoporosis (fragile bones), diabetes and an increased liability to infections. When treating lupus with steroids, the dose and duration of steroids are judged according to the degree of activity of the lupus and its implications for causing damage. Doctors looking after lupus patients are always trying to steer a course between too little steroid, resulting in active, damaging disease and too much steroid, risking excessive steroid side-effects.

There are other forms of steroid such as skin applications or for injection into joints. Betamethasone and dexamethasone are alternative tablet forms which are used in particular circumstances. An effective way of giving steroids for severe lupus is as 'pulses' or 'boluses' of large doses (500 to 1000 mgm) of methylprednisolone, almost always administered intravenously. Smaller 'mini-pulses' of 80 to 120 mgm of methylprednisolone, which can be given by intramuscular injection, may be used to control lesser flares. Some patients become very adept at identifying the dose of steroids that they individually require for good control of their lupus. Ways to minimize side-effects of steroids are discussed below and in Chapter 10.

Immunosuppressive drugs

Azathioprine and Methotrexate

While these two drugs differ from each other in terms of their chemical composition and to some extent their side-effects, they are used in rather similar fashion in the treatment of lupus. Both have to be monitored every few weeks, or more frequently depending upon dose change or blood test trends. Both can suppress resistance to infection.

Ciclosporin

This has been used principally for suppressing kidney transplants, but is sometimes useful in lupus kidney disease. It also needs monitoring, for example, for its effects on blood pressure.

Cyclophosphamide

This is a powerful immunosuppressant drug. It is **cytotoxic**, which implies that the drug can kill cells. It was developed for treating conditions such as cancer and leukaemia, because it inhibits bone marrow and other cells from multiplying. We think it works in lupus by suppressing the immune system's inappropriately vigorous production of

cytotoxic
A drug that kills cells. This usually means malignant (cancerous) cells, but in inflammatory conditions as in this book, it means the suppression or killing of cells of the immune system.

antibodies and therefore immune complexes. The details of dosage for the individual are beyond the scope of this book. For lupus it is usually given by intravenous infusion or 'bolus' – this means that it is given in a large amount in a relatively short time. Bone marrow suppression, loss of hair and lowered resistance to infection are all possible side-effects. It is only used when the lupus is likely to result in severe damage, for example, to the kidneys. It is often given in tandem with 'pulse' methylprednisolone as the combination can be very effective in controlling kidney disease. It is liable to cause damage to ovaries however.

New developments in treatment

The importance of anti-DNA antibodies in this disease has always made scientists consider that there should be a way of controlling lupus by biological means. There are possible such strategies under development. Suppression of the B cells that make antibodies with rituximab, which is used for treatment of certain cancers, is one such possibility.

Adjunctive treatment

These are methods of treating problems that may arise rather specifically in the course of lupus but which do not mean necessarily increasing the intensity of steroids or immunosuppressive drugs. Examples might include blood transfusion for anaemia, infusion of blood products such as platelets or gammaglobulin for **haematological** problems, or localized steroid injections for acute joint problems.

haematological
Blood related.

I am one of two sisters and we have one brother. Ever since I was a teenager I have suffered from chilblains and a tendency to getting tired more easily than my siblings or friends. Then when I was on holiday in Majorca with my boyfriend for my twenty-fifth birthday I became terribly sunburnt and feverish. My joints ached and swelled up. When we got home I went to my doctor who said it was just the effects of the sun. I was OK until I was 30 and working very hard in insurance sales. I developed more joint pains and swelling and felt exhausted. This time my doctor did some blood tests and found I had a positive test for 'Lupus'. I looked this up on the internet and became very scared of what might happen. I was referred to a rheumatology consultant who explained it all. I am now taking some medication that used to be used for malaria, of all things! I feel better, but am very careful to avoid the sun. I also get very tired still, but know my limitations and can cope. I am however worried about starting a family, as I recently got engaged.

Immunosuppressive drugs such as Azathioprine or methotrexate are often prescribed alongside prednisolone as a 'steroid-sparing' strategy. So, let us say that experience has shown that you need to take 20 mgm of prednisolone each day in order to control arthritis and pleuritic pains, but that is resulting in gain in weight, a puffy face and a raised blood pressure. If Azathioprine, say 100 mgm per day, is added, you might find that after a few weeks you can have the same benefit from the prednisolone at only 12.5 mgm a day. This may be enough to reduce the side-effects from the prednisolone.

My daughter became very ill with SLE (Lupus) 11 years ago at the age of 31. At first it was thought she had a urine infection and then a series of reactions to the antibiotics. It also affected her general health, with fevers and odd skin rashes. So it took nearly a year before she was diagnosed. Since then she has been in hospital five times because she has a kidney problem. We thought that we were going to lose her once, when she had fits. Fortunately these were controlled and her kidneys have stabilized. They are affected and she takes loads of tablets for blood pressure, but she is able to cope a bit better now. It is still very worrying for us though.

Q Are there any new treatments for lupus that are more effective than these old ones, or have fewer side-effects?

A Yes: there are reasonably high hopes for some new methods of treating lupus. These include:

✧ Mycophenolate mofetil – this drug was originally developed for suppressing rejection of organ transplants
✧ rituximab – this was originally used for lymphomas. It suppresses the immune B cells
✧ hormone manipulation – this includes female and male hormones
✧ immune manipulation – this is a relatively new but expanding field and includes complement modification, cytokine inhibition, stem cell therapy, and DNA antibody inhibition.

Scleroderma and systemic sclerosis

The 'sclero' bit refers to hardness or fibrosis, the 'derma' bit to skin. However, there is a lot more to it than skin involvement, so the term systemic sclerosis is used to include the fact that the fibrosis can affect internal organs such as the intestine or lungs. It is regarded as an inflammatory rheumatic disease because there is considerable evidence of inflammation, especially during the early stages of the condition. In the skin, this is manifested by puffiness (oedema), a feeling of tightness, sometimes itchiness and maybe changes in pigmentation.

Broadly, there are two main types:

✧ limited systemic sclerosis (SSc) or sclerodactyly – where the skin hardness or sclerosis is confined to the fingers

✧ diffuse SSc – where there is involvement of other tissues such as the lungs or the intestines.

There is also early involvement of small blood vessels, heralded by the development of instability of the peripheral circulation: Raynaud's phenomenon. It is those individuals with Raynaud's combined with a positive test for the ANA (see Chapter 11) who may develop SSc.

Q **My fingers feel numb and get very cold in the winter. My doctor says I have Raynaud's. I have looked it up on the Web and am worried that I might be developing scleroderma, which sounds awful. I feel quite all right generally, so how would I know if I am going to develop it?**

A First of all, having cold hands is not necessarily Raynaud's phenomenon, which means having rather unmistakeable attacks of spasm of the blood vessels of the fingers or toes (and occasionally in the ears or nose). There is a clear demarcation line between where the blood flow is normal and where the blood vessels have temporarily shut down, which is the white or purplish part, and may involve the whole finger or just the tip. There may be discomfort or tingling when the blood flow returns. Raynaud's occurs in perhaps 5 per cent of the population and SSc is much rarer, so the chances of developing SSc are low. Those people who are going to develop SSc usually have an autoantibody such as ANA in their blood at an early stage, so a negative ANA is a good and reassuring test.

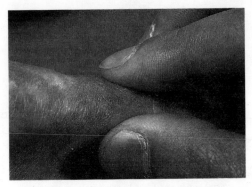

▌Figure 7.3 Loss of elasticity of the skin of the hand.

Limited systemic sclerosis

The scleroderma changes are limited to the extremities: the hands, face and feet. The damage to the skin and underlying tissue may nevertheless be quite severe, with fingertip pits and ulceration. Normally one can pinch the skin up from the back of the hand, but in scleroderma this becomes difficult because of the loss of elasticity (see figure 7.3).

The CREST syndrome is a variant of limited scleroderma. The acronym is fairly self-explanatory:

C – for Calcinosis (little deposits of calcium salts in or beneath the skin)

R – for Raynaud's

E – for Esophageal involvement (the North American spelling of Oesophageal)

S – for Sclerodactyly

T – for Telangiectasia (little spidery blood vessels on the face and hands – see plate 11).

CREST is useful shorthand for descriptive purposes, but not all the features (calcification, for

> **Q Who gets scleroderma or systemic sclerosis?**
>
> **A** It can occur at any age and in either sex, but it is four times more common in women, in whom it usually starts between the ages of 25 and 50 years.

example) are necessarily present at its onset. However, people with CREST tend also to have a positive blood test for the anti-centromere antibody, which is therefore helpful as a predictor. The oesophageal involvement causes heartburn and may result in swallowing difficulty. Rarely, lung involvement with **pulmonary hypertension** occurs.

pulmonary hypertension
Raised pressure within the lung circulation.

Q My skin has patches of dryness on it and feels different from the rest – might I have scleroderma?

A The description is not enough to be in any way certain. The diagnosis is often not easy to make. There are also skin conditions that resemble scleroderma, such as localized scleroderma, morphoea and pseudoscleroderma, where the changes are limited to patches of abnormal skin thickening. In addition there is a wide range of unusual disorders in which the skin might appear sclerodermatous, such as porphyria, organic solvent poisoning or eosinophilic fasciitis.

Systemic sclerosis

The internal organs that can be affected include:

✧ the kidney – blood vessels of the kidney are involved, producing a raised blood pressure and other damage
✧ the intestine – with diarrhoea or constipation, loss of absorptive function and weight loss
✧ the heart (cardiomyopathy) – with breathlessness and fluid retention
✧ the lungs – with breathlessness as the main feature.

Q What is the outlook for patients with scleroderma or systemic sclerosis?

A It used to be quite bleak, with kidney and lung problems causing the most severe illness and death. Medication can now control these problems to a large extent. There is also now some hope for future curative treatments, as research reveals more details of the underlying immunological abnormalities.

Treatment

Skin and circulatory problems

Since the main feature of Raynaud's is an inappropriate closing reduction in the peripheral circulation in response to cold, keeping hands and feet warm is important. Leave the house with gloved, warmed-up hands, rather than waiting for them to get cold. Avoid grasping cold objects (e.g. milk bottles from the fridge) directly and use hand warmers – available from climbers' shops. Drugs such as nifedipine can help, but may also cause headaches and ankle swelling. More intensive treatment to open up the circulation includes intravenous infusions of drugs such as prostacycline. The function of the sweat glands in the affected skin may become abnormal, so moisturizers and massage may be useful.

Heartburn

This is caused by oesophageal reflux, due to loss of normal function of the sphincter (valve) at the lower end of the oesophagus (gullet). Acid from the stomach washes up the oesophagus, causing pain and eventually the risk of scarring and blockage. Alkali medicines are usually inadequate, so a **proton pump inhibitor** such as omeprazole or a histamine H2-antagonist such as cimetidine are prescribed.

proton pump inhibitor
Reduces the acid secretions in the stomach.

Joint and tendon problems

Exercise is to be encouraged and there is no evidence that harm can be caused. Physiotherapy may help contractures. Tendon inflammation, for example, around the ankle, may benefit from local steroid injections. NSAIDs can be useful, but may have to be avoided because of oesophageal reflux.

Heart and lung problems

There are two types of lung problem: **pulmonary fibrosis** and pulmonary hypertension. Both are potentially serious complications and may occur in the same person. The normal lungs and heart, especially in young people, have considerable reserve, to allow for walking slowly to running hard. Quite a lot of this reserve lung function may be lost before someone notices they are getting breathless. People with scleroderma may not feel able to take much exercise. Therefore, they should be monitored for the development of heart or lung problems with lung function tests as well as imaging (taking pictures by X-rays, CT – computerized tomography – scanning, Spiral CT or MRI – magnetic resonance imaging).

There is increasing hope for people with these heart or lung problems. New medications are being developed which are aimed at arresting the inflammatory changes or the blood vessel problems in the lungs. This makes it even more important that these problems are identified early on, before the later irreversible scarring has time to develop.

pulmonary fibrosis
Fibrosis of the lungs.

Kidney disease and blood pressure

Drugs called ACE inhibitors were the first ones to be really effective in controlling blood pressure crises in systemic sclerosis kidney disease. Newer ones are even more effective, so monitoring blood pressure is very important.

Hints for heartburn sufferers

Avoid sleeping flat. Just using several pillows is not usually sufficient or comfortable, whereas raising the head of the bed by about 7.5 cm on blocks is helpful.

Avoid fatty foods (they slow stomach emptying); spicy foods, some fruits, tomatoes and onions are also difficult to cope with for some people.

myopathy

A muscle disorder. This can include inherited muscle disease or inflammation (myositis). It can also be caused by medication, such as prolonged treatment with high doses of steroids.

Inflammatory muscle disease: polymyositis and dermatomyositis

'Myositis' means inflammation of muscle tissue and, since a muscle's function is to produce force, the main symptom of muscle disease is loss of strength (weakness) in the affected muscles. A feeling of overall weakness is not the same thing. This can be due to fatigue, fever or other illness. Weakness of a particular muscle or muscle group can be due to a **myopathy**. This means any disease of muscle and covers all sorts of muscle problems including, for example, muscular dystrophy or high doses of steroid drugs. It does not just mean muscle pain or muscle strain. This section is confined to describing the myositis that can occur on its own or as part of a systemic rheumatic condition.

Myositis tends to affect the big muscle groups of the shoulders, upper arms, buttocks and thighs, although it can sometimes be more localized. In addition to weakness, the muscles may become wasted and tender. The enzymes found inside muscle cells leak out into the circulation, so usually this is a relatively sensitive test for the condition, provided it is suspected in the first place. Electrical tests (EMG) and a biopsy of the muscle using a needle are other investigations that are employed.

Primary polymyositis is, as its name implies, a condition that arises in the absence of anything else. 'Dermatomyositis' means that there is myositis together with a rather characteristic skin rash. Both conditions are quite rare.

Who gets dermatomyositis?

It can start in childhood or adulthood. It is more common in women than in men. It is probably an autoimmune condition and although we do not know what triggers it, there is evidence of an inappropriate immunological reaction to something, possibly an infection.

Treatment

As with other inflammatory systemic rheumatic conditions, steroids are the mainstay of treatment, often with immunosuppressants such as methotrexate to reduce the required dose of steroids. Doctors have to be aware of the problem of differentiating weakness due to the muscle disease from steroid-induced myopathy, due to high doses of prednisolone. The rash of dermatomyositis may need additional local treatment, for example, with locally applied steroid preparations or drugs such as hydroxychloroquine. Children sometimes respond well to intravenous immunoglobulin infusions.

Complications

Deposits of calcium can develop in and under the skin, similar to the calcinosis in CREST syndrome. This is probably a healing reaction to which muscle is especially liable. Contractures of the muscles are a particular problem in children with dermatomyositis and will need expert physiotherapy.

Overlap conditions

This a term used to describe patients who seem to have features of more than one systemic rheumatic disorder. For example, there may be arthritis resembling rheumatoid arthritis, together with a rash like lupus, myositis and puffy hands a bit like early scleroderma. The term mixed connective tissue disease (MCTD) was coined in the 1960s to describe such a group of symptoms. However, these are really syndromes, rather than separate diseases. That does not mean that doctors are just collecting labels like stamps, though it sometimes may seem like that! The behaviour, pattern of development, or prognosis of the collection of problems that is described with this label may be characteristic. There may also be something to be learnt scientifically, for example, when anti-DNA antibodies are absent from the blood of a patient with MCTD, then kidney disease is very unlikely to develop. The antibody profile that is characteristic of a syndrome may therefore tell us something about the precipitating cause.

Sjögren's syndrome

Sicca means dry. The term sicca syndrome is used to describe patients who have dry eyes and a dry mouth. Dr Henrich Sjögren, a Swedish ophthalmologist, originally described a group of people with the combination of dryness of the eye, due to impaired tear secretion, and arthritis. Nowadays, the term Sjögren's syndrome is used to denote patients who have the combination of the sicca syndrome together with some form of inflammatory rheumatic disease, not exclusively arthritis.

Eye symptoms of the sicca syndrome may include stickiness, filmy vision, tired eyes or grittiness. The commonest cause of a dry eye in the population is not, of course, Sjögren's syndrome. Other more likely explanations include age, medication or the menopause. Similarly, common causes of a dry mouth include sleeping with one's mouth open, smoking or anti-depressant treatment. The tear film over the surface of the eye is composed of a mucus layer, a watery (aqueous) layer and an oily layer. Probably all, but mostly the watery layer are affected by the salivary gland inflammation that characterizes Sjögren's syndrome.

Primary Sjögren's syndrome is where patients have the sicca syndrome without an additional definable rheumatic condition. However, they can develop other problems – fatigue being the most common. They may have arthralgia (joint pains) without full-blown arthritis. The salivary glands may become very swollen and painful, just like mumps. Other glands of the **exocrine** system (as distinct from the hormone glands of the **endocrine** system) may become involved. The exocrine system covers glands that secrete substances externally: for this purpose, the 'outside' can include tubes or cavities such as the mouth or the duct from the pancreas to the intestine. This contrasts with the endocrine system that secretes hormones such as thyroid hormone into the blood stream. Patients might have dry skin and hair, and vaginal dryness may be particularly troublesome. A cough results from bronchial dryness, and other chest problems may require specialist investigation. A vasculitic skin rash can occur and, rarely, neurological problems can develop. In a very small sub-group of patients with particularly severe gland involvement, there is an increase risk of lymphoma. These patients should be followed up in a specialist clinic. Other, also rare complications, of primary Sjögren's syndrome include a form of kidney disorder and liver dysfunction.

exocrine glands
These are glands that secrete substances, such as the salivary glands that make saliva.

endocrine glands
These are glands such as the thyroid or adrenal, that secrete hormones into the blood stream.

Secondary Sjögren's syndrome can develop in patients already suffering from RA. Fortunately, topical treatments such as tear supplements (see page 151) are usually sufficient to control symptoms. If sicca syndrome develops in patients with lupus or scleroderma it may be a bit more difficult to treat and may more nearly resemble the primary form.

Q My doctor says I might have Sjögren's syndrome. I've looked the symptoms up and I don't quite understand, because although my eyes feel sore, I can still feel my eyes watering sometimes, so they can't be dry. How can I find out if this is what I have? Is there a blood test?

A Yes, it does seem odd that there might be a problem with tears and yet the eyes can water. This can sometimes happen, however, when the tear film is abnormal and does not cover the eye properly and inflammation or irritation then causes excess tear production to try to compensate. Tear production is measured with a small length of filter paper. In Sjögren's syndrome it is usually reduced.

In patients with primary Sjögren's syndrome a blood test gives a positive result for antibodies to proteins called Ro and La: these are not found when Sjögren's is the secondary sort, found in association with rheumatoid arthritis. If there is still doubt as to whether you have Sjögren's syndrome, the doctors may advise that a biopsy is taken of your salivary gland. This sounds a bit frightening but, fortunately, tissue does not have to be taken from your parotid gland (the one in front of the ear that swells up in mumps). Saliva is also made by the little glands that are dotted all over the lining membrane of your mouth. A very small piece of tissue from the back of your lip is taken under local anaesthetic and examined under a microscope. The only risk with this is a slight, temporary, numbness of the lip.

Treatment

Topical treatments

Tear substitutes of various types are widely available at the pharmacy. People with sicca syndrome may need to put the drops in very frequently – maybe every couple of hours. A commonly used active constituent is methylcellulose. The preservative added to it may irritate the eye, so it is best to use preservative-free drops, keep the tube or bottle in the fridge and discard it every month, even if it is unfinished. A long acting ointment substitute can be helpful for night-time use.

In resistant cases, little plugs can be put in the tear duct that emerges at the inner corner of the eye. This is a minor procedure and can be reversed.

There are no satisfactory ways of replacing saliva. A drug called pilocarpine increases salivary flow, but can cause uncomfortable flushing or other side-effects.

Systemic treatment

Hydroxychloroquine may be helpful in relatively mild cases, to alleviate fatigue, joint pain or skin rashes. In more severe cases, especially if there are any complications as mentioned above, steroids are used, with or without methotrexate or azathioprine. In very severe cases, the approach is similar to that for severe lupus or vasculitis.

The outlook for patients with Sjögren's syndrome is, on the whole, positive as it is not a serious disorder in terms of risk of serious illness or death. There are exceptions, but most of the problems can be controlled as outlined above.

Tips

The following tips may help to alleviate symptoms:

✧ avoid dry, dusty or smoke-filled environments
✧ turn down the central heating or use a humidifier
✧ always carry a small bottle of water
✧ avoid bright sunlight
✧ stop smoking
✧ ensure regular dental check-ups
✧ don't chew sugary confectionary
✧ discuss any medication with your doctor to ensure it is unlikely to make the dryness worse
✧ consult an optician if you have contact lenses – you may have to discontinue them, but some are specially designed to reduce evaporation.

Systemic vasculitis

The term 'vasculitis' refers to the blood vessel inflammation that can occur in conditions such as RA or SLE. This in itself is quite uncommon. Systemic vasculitis is even more infrequent.

There is a wide range of symptoms but the patient generally feels unwell, usually with a fever, and experiences sweats, fatigue and weight loss. Specific symptoms might include joint pain, abdominal pain, chest problems, kidney disease, numbness or weakness due to nerve inflammation or skin rashes with ulceration.

The following are most of the different types of vasculitis:

✧ giant cell arteritis: (described on page 157, with polymyalgia rheumatica)

✧ Wegener's granulomatosis (particularly involves the lungs, the kidney, the mucosal linings of the nose and sinuses)

✧ Churg-Strauss disease (particularly gives rise to a type of asthma, nerve inflammation and heart problems)

✧ polyarteritis nodosa (especially the kidneys, nerves and skin)

✧ microscopic polyangiitis (principally kidney problems)

✧ Kawasaki disease (causes glandular swelling and occasionally heart inflammation in children)

✧ Takayasu's arteritis (this is sometimes called 'pulseless' disease, because it affects the large blood vessels such as the aorta)

✧ Henoch-Schönlein Purpura (skin, kidney and intestines).

These names have arisen over the years, initially by virtue of their differing clinical symptoms. More recently the underlying similarities have become apparent but the various types are still worth distinguishing by some differences in pathological features, such as the appearance on biopsy of affected tissue or the size of the blood vessels affected, as well as antibodies found in the blood. At first sight the descriptions make the vasculitic conditions seem rather like the wide range of problems found in SLE. However, there are very important differences in the nature of the underlying disease processes and causes.

It will be apparent that many people affected by these conditions have no arthritis or other rheumatic symptoms. They may be looked after by kidney specialists (nephrologists), respiratory physicians or ear nose and throat consultants. There is, however, usually good research and clinical collaboration between specialists who have particular expertise in the same area of medicine. So, for example, nephrologists and rheumatologists may collaborate on treatment trials of new drugs or combinations of drugs in the treatment of vasculitis, such as Wegener's, affecting the kidneys.

Q Who gets systemic vasculitis?

A It can occur at any age, but people of different ages tend to be affected by different types of vasculitis. For example, Henoch-Schönlein Purpura and Kawasaki disease are more likely to affect children. Giant cell arteritis, which occurs as an extension of the much more common polymyalgia rheumatica, is extremely unusual under the age of 50. Vasculitis in general is a bit more likely in older people than is lupus. There are around 3000 new cases of vasculitis in the UK each year: this excludes all the cases of polymyalgia rheumatica. There are some geographical variations in the types and frequencies of vasculitis across the world: Takayasu's arteritis, for example, is much commoner in Asia and Japan than in Europe.

Q How is vasculitis diagnosed?

A The first clue is from the patient's history and then the clinical features on examination, for example, a characteristic rash that differs from those in lupus. The pattern of involvement (e.g. lungs + kidney + skin) is an important guide to diagnosis.

Blood tests are very useful: in lupus, the ANA and its related tests are positive, whereas in vasculitis the **ANCA** test, with similar related tests, is positive. In Churg-Strauss syndrome there is a

ANCA (anti-neutrophil cytoplasmic antibody)
Antibody found in patients with systemic vasculitis.

rise in the eosinophil cells of the blood; these are generally associated with allergies, hence the theory that this type of vasculitis is an exaggerated hypersensitivity to something like an infection or a drug. A biopsy of the affected tissue, such as the kidney, nasal sinuses or skin, is often the decisive test.

Symptoms of vasculitis

The skin

A purple-ish blotchy rash is usual on the skin, which may crust over or ulcerate (see figure 7.4). The rash of Henoch-Schönlein Purpura, usually in children, consists of discrete blotches which last for several days.

The nervous system

Pins and needles, numbness and weakness due to nerve damage can all occur, especially in the Churg-Strauss type. Brain involvement is, however, very rare.

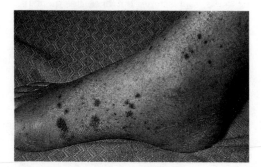

Figure 7.4 A vasculitis rash on the foot.

The kidney

Any of the types may involve the kidney, but it is especially characteristic of Wegener's and Polyangiitis. Early signs of kidney disease often go unnoticed, so if vasculitis is suspected because of, for example, the skin rash, then tests for kidney function should be carried out at once.

The lungs and respiratory tract

Wegener's characteristically affects the sinuses, producing bleeding, crusting, pain and blockage. This may at first be thought to be just severe sinusitis, but the severity and presence of bleeding are important indications of vasculitis.

The eyes

There can be inflammation of the eye in the form of conjunctivitis, or swelling of the eye because of collections of the **granulomatous** material behind it.

granulomatous
A type of chronic inflammation.

The joints

Arthritis is quite common in, for example, Wegener's or Henoch-Schönlein Purpura. It can be quite troublesome, but once treatment has become established to suppress the vasculitis, long-term damage as in RA is unlikely.

Treatment

Some cases of vasculitis are triggered by infection, for example, hepatitis viruses. Drugs have been incriminated in other cases. However, that does not mean that all cases are caused by either drugs or infection. The term 'granulomatous' is used to describe the nature of the pathology seen under the microscope on a biopsy. This granulomatous appearance resembles that of chronic infections, involving **neutrophils** and other phagocytic cells that digest bacteria. Just treating vasculitis with antibiotics does not work. However, especially when the sinuses are involved, as they often are in the syndrome called Wegener's granulomatosis, there may be some advantage in treating or preventing infection.

Other specific problems such as anaemia or pain can be treated in a way similar to that described for inflammatory arthritis or lupus. A regimen that involves a combination of steroid drugs (prednisolone or similar) and an immunosuppressive drug, such as cyclophosphamide, methotrexate or azathioprine, is almost always required to bring the active condition under control. Very often a similar combination, in modified dosage, is required for maintenance. Intravenous immunoglobulin is useful for Kawasaki disease and sometimes other types.

Polymyalgia rheumatica (PMR)

This is the characteristic story of a patient with polymyalgia rheumatica (PMR), who is rather more likely to be female than male, will be at least 50 years old – and very likely to be quite a lot older.

The patient will start feeling extremely stiff around the shoulders and perhaps the hips as well. She will struggle to raise her arms above shoulder level to dress and will have difficulty in turning over in bed. She may feel unwell, a bit feverish and lose her appetite. If she consults her doctor, the diagnosis will be suspected, as it is quite a characteristic picture.

neutrophils
A white cell subtype.

Q What is the outlook for a patient with vasculitis?

A That very much depends upon the individual situation, the tissues affected, how early the diagnosis is made and how soon effective treatment can be started. The use of drug regimes involving cyclophosphamide has made a significant difference, but we cannot be complacent: this is a serious condition, which needs to be taken seriously.

A blood test will reveal:

✧ slight anaemia, but no sign of iron deficiency
✧ a raised ESR, to over 50 mm per hour.

The doctor will then prescribe prednisolone in a dose of 20 mgm per day. Within one week there will be very considerable improvement; the dose of steroid will be reduced after a bit longer, but maintained for over one year before it can be withdrawn without a relapse. The doctor will ensure that the patient will at least take adequate calcium and Vitamin D, but may prescribe a bisphosphonate as well, to ward off osteoporosis induced by the steroid.

That is in some ways the ideal situation. However, not every case proceeds as satisfactorily. The diagnosis may not be straightforward or it may prove difficult to withdraw the steroids without a relapse. Some patients have to take steroids for years, perhaps in a dose as small as 3–5 mgm

Q **I feel awfully stiff around the shoulders. My doctor said he thought I had developed polymyalgia rheumatica, but now says I cannot be suffering from it because my erythrocyte sedimentation rate is normal. How can that be? A friend of mine had the same symptoms and did very well on steroids. Why can't I be treated with this drug?**

A There are several causes of stiffness around the shoulders. Usually these can be diagnosed clinically (see Chapter 3). If it is not one of these, it is still possible to have PMR with a normal ESR, although it is unusual. In this case, a trial of treatment with prednisolone can be done, but there must be a convincing benefit within a week or so to a dose of around 20 mgm of prednisolone daily. Neither the patient nor the doctor should be led by default into prolonged treatment with steroids without a secure diagnosis.

prednisolone a day. Some people need a dose of 10 mgm a day or more to suppress pain and stiffness, but then start to get steroid side-effects. In those cases, a drug such as azathioprine may be added as a 'steroid-sparing' agent, to maintain suppression of inflammation with a smaller dose of steroid.

Complications of PMR

A small proportion of patients with PMR develop giant cell arteritis at about the same time or later. These patients will require a much higher dose of prednisolone (see below) to prevent blindness. So all patients with PMR should report immediately to their doctor if they develop scalp tenderness, a sudden unusual headache or blurring of vision.

The other complications of PMR are mostly to do with steroid treatment (see Chapter 10 for further details).

Giant cell arteritis (GCA)

Giant cell arteritis (GCA) is also known as cranial arteritis or temporal arteritis. It consists of inflammation in an artery of the scalp, such as the temporal artery at the temple. Sometimes other arteries, such as the occipital one at the back of the skull, are involved. The internal arteries of the brain may also be involved, but the one most likely is an artery to the eye. There is accumulation of so-called 'giant cells' in the artery, often quite patchily. The sufferer develops intense headache and pain with tenderness and often swelling and redness over the affected blood vessel. Wearing spectacles or brushing the hair may be very painful.

GCA can arise with no other symptoms. However, more often it develops in patients who also have PMR. Whichever is the case, high doses of steroids are needed to control inflammation and prevent the most feared complication – blindness in one or even both eyes.

The diagnosis is suspected clinically, but almost always an attempt is made to take a biopsy of a suspect artery, if accessible. It is preferable to do this before steroids are started, but it may be considered more important to get going with the steroid treatment as soon as the diagnosis is made with no further delay.

CHAPTER

8

Arthritis and infection

Many infections can affect the joints. If the infective organism gets inside the joint it is called **septic arthritis**. If it causes an illness during which inflammation of the joints develops, it is termed *reactive* or *infection-associated* arthritis. This is an important difference. The term 'infectious arthritis' is sometimes taken to mean septic arthritis and sometimes to describe reactive arthritis, so it is not used at all here.

Unfortunately there are some other terminological problems. The term 'reactive arthritis' is sometimes reserved for Reiter's syndrome, which may be caused by the dysentery organism Shigella or by Salmonella. People who happen to have inherited the HLA B27 gene are peculiarly susceptible to this condition (see Chapter 5, page 93).

However, there is a wide range of types of other infections, during or following which an inflammatory arthritis may develop. Everyone is

> **septic arthritis**
> An infection of a joint by a bacterium. Reactive or infection-associated arthritis is arthritis developing because of an infection, but where the organism is not actually found in the joint.

familiar with the aching in muscles and joints that can occur with infections such as influenza. However, there are more clearly defined arthritic conditions that can occur as a result of infections, not necessarily during the active infection itself. They do not happen very often and they have no characteristic features in common with each other, but the possibility of such a situation should be considered whenever anyone becomes ill with a fever and/or a rash and then develops joint pains.

Septic arthritis

In septic arthritis there are infective organisms – bacteria – inside the joint. It is closely related to osteomyelitis, where the bug is in the bone, so these are discussed together. The bacterium most frequently involved is the staphylococcus, but others occur. People who are susceptible to septic arthritis are mostly, but not entirely, those with developing or weakened immune systems such as:

✧ children
✧ the elderly
✧ the malnourished
✧ the immune-compromised (e.g. on immunosuppressive drugs)
✧ those with abnormal joints:
 – with joints damaged by inflammatory arthritis
 – with penetrating injuries of joints
 – with artificial materials in their joints (arthroplasties or injury with foreign bodies).

The term 'penetrating injury' can of course include medical interference, such as with a needle – hence the efforts taken to avoid this (see Chapter 10). When tuberculosis (TB) was a common problem in the UK, TB of the joints or bone was unfortunately all too often a complication. It remains a scourge in developing countries and is showing signs of re-emergence here, so no one can be complacent. It is also a complication of HIV infection.

Suspecting and diagnosing septic arthritis

To diagnose septic arthritis requires the suspicion of it. A toddler who refuses to try to walk; an elderly man with known osteoarthritis (OA) who becomes drowsy, feverish and has even more difficulty than usual in walking; a patient with rheumatoid arthritis (RA) who says that one of her joints is very painful, but that it feels different from a flare of her arthritis. All these and indeed anyone with an acutely inflamed hot, red, painful joint should be taken seriously as possible candidates for having septic arthritis. To make the diagnosis requires taking a sample of fluid with a needle from the suspected joint and sending it off, urgently, to a laboratory for testing. There it will be cultured to grow the organism, so that it can be more precisely identified and so that the antibiotic most likely to be effective can be chosen.

Pseudo gout

This inflammatory complication of an osteoarthritic joint (Chapter 2) is caused by crystals of **pyrophosphate**, which can also produce fever. I am mentioning it here because it tends to occur in elderly people and therefore can be confused with septic arthritis. The fluid that is removed can look

pyrophosphate
A chemical substance that occurs normally throughout the body. However, especially with advancing age, it may accumulate in joint cartilage as crystals. These can sometimes cause inflammation. This may be acute or similar to gout – hence the term 'pseudo-gout'. Or a rather more grumbling inflammation may develop.

like pus because pus consists of millions of white blood cells (polymorphonuclear leucocytes). These will respond to crystals in the same way that they respond to bacteria: by trying to engulf and digest them. In the process, loads of inflammatory molecules are released. These cause redness, pain and swelling that characterize an abscess or pustule. The diagnosis requires fluid to be extracted from the joint and sent to a laboratory to be examined under the polarizing microscope.

Types of reactive or infection-associated arthritis

myth
Rheumatic fever no longer exists.

fact
Rheumatic fever is rare in the UK, but is more common overseas and can affect people coming to this country. Streptococcal infection can cause arthritis.

Infections that can affect the joints, without infecting them, include:

- ✧ rheumatic fever
- ✧ streptococcal infections
- ✧ rubella (German measles)
- ✧ Parvovirus B19 ('Slapped Cheek Syndrome' or 'Fifth Disease')
- ✧ mumps
- ✧ chlamydia
- ✧ gonococcus
- ✧ Shigella
- ✧ Salmonella
- ✧ yersinia
- ✧ campylobacter
- ✧ hepatitis B
- ✧ hepatitis C
- ✧ HIV.

Rheumatic fever and streptococcal arthritis

The most well known of these, at least to an older generation, is rheumatic fever. This is an idiosyncratic reaction to infection with the streptococcus organism. In the earlier parts of the twentieth century it was very common in the UK, leading to many deaths from heart complications (carditis). Even if the person did not die, they were often left with damage to the valves of the heart. In fact it was mostly these patients who were the early people to be treated with cardiac surgery, by replacing damaged heart valves with artificial ones. The arthritis was usually not very severe. It tended to flit from one joint to another, often within a few hours. It did not produce the same joint damage as RA, but could leave a rather similar and characteristic deformity of the fingers. In the 1930s, even before penicillin came into use, the frequency of rheumatic fever began to fall, probably as housing started to improve and the importance of public health was recognized more widely. We can never become complacent about infections, however, and rheumatic fever is found elsewhere in the world, so no one can be assumed to be immune. Interestingly, we rheumatologists get the impression that there is a type of mild arthritis associated with streptococcal infection such as sore throats. It is a sort of *forme fruste* of rheumatic fever and does not affect the heart.

Rubella (German measles)

Most people are familiar with rubella and are aware of its potential for producing problems in the fetus if a pregnant woman becomes infected with rubella. Hence the policy of immunization for girls. A type of inflammatory arthritis may develop directly from infection; in fact there is some evidence that the virus may grow inside the joint, setting up the inflammation. This is not a common problem, since rubella is itself not common nowadays, but it can still occur. The arthritis occurs more often in younger adults than in children, so should be remembered as a possible explanation when a young women develops swollen and painful joints. A blood test usually distinguishes between recent infection and previous immunization. The arthritis may last for several months and require treatment with anti-inflammatory medication.

Parvovirus

Parvovirus B19 is the type of Parvovirus bug that can cause an arthritis. Similarly to the rubella instance, children who develop this infection usually just have the illness, which can produce the bright red cheek that gives it the name of Slapped Cheek Syndrome. An adult (such as a parent or teacher of young children) may develop an inflammatory arthritis without the red cheek, so once again one must suspect it as a possible diagnosis. It will usually settle down after a few weeks or months.

Mumps

As we are seeing a reduced protection of the population because of concerns over triple vaccination, we might see more cases of this unusual complication of mumps. And perhaps we shall see it in young adults rather than children, by analogy with rubella.

Chlamydia

This predominantly genital infection is not well known as a cause of arthritis, but it can be quite troublesome and chronic. The arthritis has no particular diagnostic features, although it tends to affect only a few joints. The infecting organism is not easily identifiable within the joint fluid, but the genital infection can and should be treated with antibiotics. So again it is important to suspect it and carry out the appropriate tests. Males and females can develop it, almost always as young adults.

Gonococcus

As with chlamydia, if any young adult develops inflammatory arthritis rather rapidly, the gonococcus must be suspected. The social history and sexual contacts have to be considered. The gonococcus can produce quite an acute illness with a rash; the gonococcus organism can be grown from the blood or the joint fluid, or an inflammatory arthritis may develop a week or two after the acute illness.

Shigella and Salmonella

The arthritis that results from these is discussed under spondylarthropathies in Chapter 5 (page 96), because it has certain clinical and genetic characteristics.

Yersinia and campylobacter

Yersinia is an unusual infection in the UK, but is more common elsewhere, especially in northern Europe and the USA. The infection can be quite severe and consists of fever, diarrhoea, abdominal pain and vomiting. If an attack of arthritis results, it comes on after the acute infection settles down, even if it is treated successfully with antibiotics. Campylobacter infection is more common and the organism is more widespread. The illness is often quite a mild form of diarrhoea and the arthritis that follows in less than 1 per cent of infections is also mild and self-limiting.

Hepatitis B, hepatitis C and HIV – AIDS

These are clustered together, not because they are unimportant, but because cases of arthritis due to these infections have no special characteristics and must be suspected from other clues. For example, if a young man rapidly becomes ill with painful swollen joints the suspicion of hepatitis should be raised even if he is not jaundiced. If someone is HIV positive, especially if AIDS has developed, he or she is more susceptible than average to develop infections of various sorts, including bacterial infections of joints. A type of arthritis resembling psoriatic arthritis appears to be more common in AIDS patients.

CHAPTER

9

Bone conditions

This is a book about arthritis, so it is not primarily about bone itself, important though it is as part of a joint. However, there are three bone conditions that can be usefully covered, albeit briefly. This does not mean that they are unimportant, but that they only impinge upon arthritis in an indirect way. They are:

- ✧ osteoporosis
- ✧ osteomalacia
- ✧ Paget's disease.

Osteoporosis

Osteoporosis has been mentioned in Chapter 5 and patients with rheumatoid arthritis (RA) are liable to develop it because they are quite likely also to be female, post-menopausal, physically inactive and on steroids. Such stereotypes are anathema to some, but they are useful reminders. If steroid treatment is considered the only or main risk factor, it would be referred to as secondary osteoporosis, but often there are multiple causes.

Strictly speaking, the word *osteopenia* should be applied to people with a specified degree of bone thinning. Osteoporosis is then reserved for people with a greater degree of bone loss and an enhanced risk of, or actual experience of, low-impact fracture. So osteopenia may lead to frank osteoporosis. In broad terms, osteoporosis means that the density and mechanical strength of the bones is less than it should be, so that there is an increased risk of fracture. One in three women and one in twelve men are likely to have an osteoporotic fracture by the age of 90. Osteoporotic fractures are usually of the wrist, the hip or the spine. They are a common and increasing cause of disability in the elderly and infirm. This is due to a number of factors, including:

◇ oestrogen deficiency – especially with an early menopause (before the age of 45)
◇ testosterone deficiency
◇ physical inactivity and weak muscles
◇ advancing years
◇ family history
◇ steroid treatment.

Osteopenia and osteoporosis are not themselves painful, so patients do not know that their bones are thin until they have had a painful fracture. The stooped posture of an elderly lady (or man) is most often due to osteoporosis affecting the spine (see figure 9.1). There are no unequivocal blood tests yet available for widespread use, so the mineral and structural content of a bone has to be measured by a bone density scan, using one of a number of different technologies.

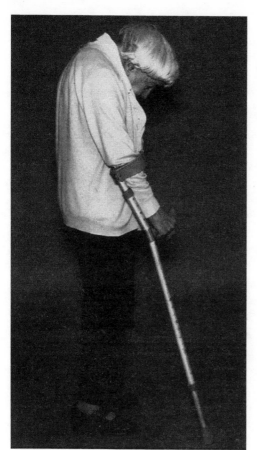

I noticed that my mother was becoming more stooped as she was getting into her 70s. She broke her wrist when she was about 68 and I thought all this was just what happens with age. However, one day I was with her in her kitchen when she tried to lift up the lower sash window. She let out a cry of pain and couldn't move because of the pain in the middle of her back. I got her to hospital where they said she had broken one of the bones in her spine. It took over a month for the pain to settle down properly and now she is on tablets to try to prevent the same thing happening again.

Figure 9.1 Elderly lady with stoop due to spinal osteoporosis.

Treatment may be based upon a known risk, for example, if someone has had a fracture from a minor fall, or if they are liable to be taking steroids for a long time. A scan is not an essential step before commencing treatment for osteoporosis, but may be requested in order to measure the effect of treatment or if there is doubt about the necessity for treatment.

The mainstay of treatment is currently one of

the bisphosphonate drugs, such as risedronate and alendronate, but they can cause stomach upsets and other side-effects. Since they act slowly, they may be given weekly or even less often. It is possible that once-yearly infusions into a vein may be effective. It is also worth remembering that dietary calcium and vitamin D deficiency are quite common in elderly people, contributing to bone weakness. Fractures are caused by falls, so unsteadiness (for example due to medication or dizziness) is also a problem contributing to fracture risk.

Osteomalacia

This is due to deficiency of vitamin D in adults. It is the adult equivalent of childhood rickets. As a dietary deficiency, rickets is fortunately now rare in the UK although it can develop in certain metabolic or kidney disorders. In adults, deficiency of vitamin D, producing osteomalacia, can be due to kidney disease or dietary deficiency and is worth remembering as a possible cause of aches and pains, mimicking arthritis. Susceptible people include elderly people whether living at home or in institutions, because they do not get enough sunlight and may live on a vitamin-deficient diet. Asian people, especially if vegans, are quite often found to suffer from this. In sunny countries sunlight on the skin allows people to make sufficient vitamin D, but a move to the UK may result in deficiency.

Osteomalacia is usually quite easy to test for and to diagnose, but it must be suspected first. The symptoms include general fatigue, muscle pain, weakness and also bone pain. X-rays are almost diagnostic as little fractures in bone can be seen. Blood tests for calcium and vitamin D levels are able to confirm the clinical suspicion in most cases. Very occasionally the removal of a tiny piece of bone for analysis (bone biopsy) is necessary.

Paget's disease

This is a disease of the bones, which become distorted. The affected bone becomes thicker, but also weaker. This may cause no symptoms at all, and may be only detected by chance. This might be when an X-ray is taken for another symptom such as back pain. Or it may be picked up when a blood test is done for some other reason, since it causes an increase in the blood level of an enzyme called alkaline phosphatase. This enzyme is included as part of the group of tests for liver function.

Paget's disease may cause pain when it affects a bone near a joint, because it can cause a type of osteoarthritis. If it affects the skull it can cause deformity and pressure on parts of the nervous system. Occasionally it causes pain or discomfort over the affected part, such as the thigh. Deformity of the shin bone can develop. Rarely it can lead to other more serious problems, even a very rare type of cancer. Many, perhaps most, patients with Paget's disease require no treatment, but complications such as fractures can occur. So sometimes the level of alkaline phosphatase or other blood tests are repeated at intervals to see if the levels are rising. If this is the case, the condition is probably active. If this is bad enough to give rise to symptoms, it can be treated with one of the bisphosphonates drugs.

CHAPTER

10

Treatment – and what to expect

Arthritis varies in its impact on a person. Perhaps no treatment at all is necessary, except an appreciation of what the symptoms mean and then an acceptance of them. Or maybe an alteration in lifestyle, ambitions or circumstances will do the trick. If treatment is required, need it consist of medication, with all the attendant risks? And if drugs or other treatments are recommended to control the condition, what are these risks, how can they be minimized and how different will the outcome be?

Throughout this chapter the reader should bear in mind the old medico-scientific adage:

'Lack of evidence of effect is not the same thing as evidence of lack of effect.'

Clinical trials are enormously expensive to set up and pharmaceutical companies can only be expected to fund studies of the products from which they make a living (as do their employees). No one is ever completely neutral about their own products or indeed their own research and this chapter cannot be free of bias either, although every effort has been made to survey the area in a reasonably objective manner.

Lifestyle

It is surely worthwhile considering the possibility that your lifestyle is relevant to your arthritis, at least in some way. From gout to fibromyalgia, back pain to tennis elbow, lupus to rheumatoid arthritis (RA), there are aspects of an individual's life and circumstances that bear upon their symptoms and how they cope with them. The following discussion takes them in no particular order of importance.

Exercise and rest

Arthritis and rheumatism are problems of the organs and systems of locomotion and physical function. Almost no matter what type or the degree of severity of the problem, exercise will help retain as much of these faculties as possible. This may require involvement of a health professional, but a great deal can be done by the individual. The matter of body weight and its effect on the normal functioning of joints has been touched upon in Chapter 2, but is worth reiterating. Joints do not wear out under normal loads and circumstances, but all tissues have a finite limit as to how far they can bear heavy impacts or repetitious use, while retaining the ability to compensate or recover. If they are exposed progressively to loads, they can respond by accommodating such loads up to a limit.

> **quotation**
> *"Those who think that they have not time for bodily exercise will sooner or later have to find time for illness."* Edward Stanley (1799–1869), 14th Earl of Derby

Many people maintain that they are 'kept busy'. Walking to the shops, vacuuming or ironing are all activities, but it is tempting to abandon them if they prove difficult or painful. Manual labour is much less widespread than in days gone by, so if a real change in physical exertion is to take place, it must be managed and planned. This may require an alteration in habits, such as walking to work, taking the stairs instead of the lift and going for real exertional walks. Heart and lungs permitting, which may mean an endorsement from your doctor, this means being willing and determined to get out of breath. Briefly, your pulse rate and rate of recovery from exercise is a guide to your ability to cope with exercise. There is no point (and some risk) in exercising until your heart is pounding, you feel faint and if it takes you hours to recover.

myth
Modern medicines are safe.

fact
There can be no absolute certainty of safety, nor absolute certainty of benefit, from any medicine.

my experience

About 12 years ago, when I was in my 40s, I started to get trouble with my joints. I would describe it as more of a persisting discomfort rather than a pain. I thought it would pass and just got on with my busy business life. There was very little swelling but the problem became rather disturbing so after about two years I consulted my doctor. He thought I had arthritis and referred me to a rheumatologist. He agreed and diagnosed rheumatoid arthritis. The ESR (erythrocyte sedimentation rate) test was somewhat raised and the Rheumatoid Factor test was positive. I started taking Plaquenil. This did not settle the symptoms, so Sulfasalazine was added. The symptoms became worse and I was prescribed ibuprofen as well as the others.

As the dose of ibuprofen was increased it started to upset my stomach, so it was swapped for Vioxx. Unfortunately this drug caused bleeding in my stools.

Vioxx was taken off the market. As an alternative, the rheumatologist then suggested that I should start treatment with Methotrexate, in place of the Sulfasalazine and Plaquenil. At the time I was working hard and travelling a lot both in the UK and to other countries such as the USA and China. I couldn't see how I could fit all the blood tests and so forth into my life as well as work. I decided therefore not to go this route and stayed with the Sulfasalazine and Plaquenil using Co-codamol for pain relief.

After having the symptoms for about four years my feet started to become very painful and I experienced a lot of discomfort in my legs particularly around the knee area. I consulted a podiatrist who prescribed some special insoles for my shoes. This improved things considerably. After dropping the Vioxx my feet were becoming particularly painful again. In fact at one point it was thought I had gout as well as rheumatoid! I consulted a podiatrist again. She said I needed major adjustments in the geometry of the special insoles for my shoes and also advised me to do lots of stretching exercises for the tendons and joints in my legs and feet. The combination of new insoles and the exercises made a vast improvement.

I was also rather overweight and my blood pressure had increased significantly. My wife and I decided that together we should make a real effort to lose weight and take more exercise. We started going to the gym and doing lots of walking. We also ate (and drank!) more healthily. I took no particular vitamins, food supplements, or remedies, apart from the prescribed medications.

I bought some good quality, well-fitting trainers and walking boots that could accommodate my insoles for exercising in the gym and walking.

Over the next nine months or so I lost three stones in weight. My wife and I worked hard at exercise, going to the gym or doing hill walks. I can say with certainty that my arthritis has progressively improved. I still take Sulfasalazine and Plaquenil, but I rarely need painkillers. My ESR is in single figures and the Rheumatoid Factor has diminished. I feel healthy and my blood pressure has come down. The stretching has been especially helpful for my legs and feet.

All this improvement has also coincided with retirement. However, I believe that it just shows how it is not one factor that controls arthritis, but a mixture of healthy living and exercise, together with medication when really necessary. In fact there is a real possibility that I will be able to stop my medication soon.

Load-bearing exercise is potentially a real problem for people with arthritis of the hips, knees or feet. Exercise in water is one answer and it doesn't have to be the Dead Sea, although that might be a wonderful way to do it! Even if you cannot swim, exercise is still possible in a pool. If you are unwilling to expose yourself to the public gaze, it is usually possible to find a pool or health club with closed sessions. Supervised hydrotherapy is a finite resource and therefore not readily available without a medical referral, but can be especially helpful for back problems and walking difficulties. Land-based exercise regimes such as modified keep fit classes, t'ai chi, Pilates and yoga are all practical possibilities for the arthritic person. The stretching and balance required for some of these is particularly helpful for stiff joints and spines.

Patients with active inflammatory disease will often feel exhausted and seek bed rest. This may be very restorative and for some people regular periods of rest are essential. However, it is important to get the disease under control with treatment, rather than to hope that it will settle by itself. Prolonged bed rest is unwise, especially for patients with advanced arthritis, who may quite quickly develop contractures. So the temptation to put pillows under painful knees should be resisted (see figure 10.1). If you sleep apparently deeply for long periods but awake still feeling tired, then this is not restorative sleep and you should be asking why – anxiety is the likely cause. Sleep interrupted by pain is a matter that needs addressing by treating joint pain.

There is a range of statutory health and social services agencies from which help may be available, depending upon the degree of dependency. The first line of help should be your

myth
Modern medicines are safer because they have been designed properly, compared with herbal stuff that might poison you.

fact
Many modern medicines are derived from herbs. Examples include: aspirin, digoxin, the contraceptive pill and several anti-cancer drugs. However, the active constituents have been refined and concentrated, so as to be more powerful and predictable.

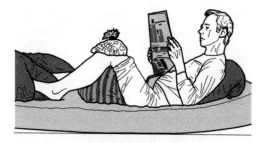

❚ Figure 10.1 Try to avoid resting like this.

doctor and team. Modification of the home and provision of aids may be necessary and the occupational therapy team will advise on this.

Diet, herbal and complementary medical products

Weight reduction has been discussed earlier and there are few overweight people who cannot lose weight if they actually eat less and better, while exercising more. For these few who have not managed to do so, there are medical avenues such as medication and stomach staple procedures but discussion of these is beyond the scope of this book.

When it comes to considering special diets or dietary supplements for the arthritic, the choices are legion. There is far more opinion than evidence and there are many people queuing up to take your money. The market for this sector of products grew by 45 per cent between 1999 and 2004.

Some dietary constituents are analogous to the non-steroidal anti-inflammatory drugs (NSAIDs), in reducing inflammation in a mild and non-specific way. Others might, at a pinch, be regarded as a bit like the disease-modifying anti-rheumatic drugs

> **myth**
> Herbal products are natural and therefore safe.

> **fact**
> This statement is partly true, but you could also describe belladonna (Deadly Nightshade) as a natural herb – and look what that can do to you!

(DMARDs), of the pharmaceutical approaches, discussed below and elsewhere in Chapters 5 and 7.

Fish oils

There is persuasive evidence that fish oils contain anti-inflammatory fatty acids, which can reduce the release of pro-inflammatory mediator molecules such as leucotrienes and interleukins. They act as precursors for anti-inflammatory prostaglandins, which inhibit platelet aggregation and other inflammatory events. In inflammatory conditions such as RA and systemic lupus erythematosus (SLE) this effect appears to be clinically detectable. We therefore now have a base of evidence that enables us to recommend their use. It is more difficult to be able to say with certainty how much, how often and for how long. Anything over 10 g per day is unlikely to be palatable enough to be sustainable, even if it were recommended. A more practical aim would be between 2 and 6 g of fish oil daily, containing the Omega-3 fatty acids eicosapentaenoic (EPA), decosahexaenoic or docosapentanoic acids. These are found in cod liver oil, herring, mackerel, salmon and sardines. There are also concentrations of such fatty acids in seal oils and palm oils.

This is a complex area of dietary science and it is easy to become over-enthusiastic about the effects of such 'natural' products. Laboratory evidence of anti-inflammatory effects in laboratory conditions does not necessarily mean that there are benefits for healthy humans, or for humans with inflammatory diseases. The ethics of killing large quantities of endangered species in order to extract oils to give to human beings, with or without good reason, is another question.

myth
Complementary medicines are more effective than conventional medicines.

fact
Very few complementary medicines have been exposed to vigorous clinical trial. So the evidence that they work is mostly lacking. However, provided that there is a combination of long established use, identifiable content and reputable retailing, then safety is more or less assured.

Selenium

Selenium is a trace mineral that is involved in anti-oxidant production in the body. Its deficiency has been associated with chronic disorders of the immune system such as unusual forms of thyroid deficiency. There have been reports of low blood levels in arthritis. However, once again one should interpret such evidence with caution. A low intake of selenium may lead to disease, but that deficiency has to be gross for such disease to occur. And this phenomenon does not necessarily imply that low blood levels in arthritic patients mean that these levels are causative, or that 'restoring' them will improve arthritis.

Copper

Copper bracelets have been used by arthritis sufferers for millennia. There are some bits of scientific research that might make one consider that there may be an argument in favour, such as the interactions of copper with immunoglobulins. Copper is probably absorbed from bracelets, since they make one's wrist green. However, trials that have involved copper supplements have been unconvincing. There is therefore no evidence that supplementing a balanced diet with copper is helpful or indeed, safe. A bracelet, however, is at least safe!

Magnetism

Magnetism has been a source of fascination for centuries. It seems rational that such a powerful, natural, but invisible influence should be able to be harnessed as a force for good. The trouble is, there is again no evidence that this is so. The enormously powerful magnetic fields involved in magnetic resonance imaging (MRI) have so far been shown to have no biological effects whatever, so it seems a little unlikely that a tiny magnet, however stylish, worn on one's wrist is likely to do anything at all. A recent medical journal summarized the position thus: 'clinically ineffective, financially harmful'.

Dehydroepiandrosterone

Dehydroepiandrosterone (DHEA) is a steroid hormone, related to the sex hormones oestrogen and testosterone. Claims have been made for its efficacy in many disorders, including several rheumatic ones. It certainly has biological effects, but they may not be desirable. It would be unwise to take this hormone without reliable medical input.

Green-lipped mussels

Green-lipped mussel extracts do have laboratory evidence in their favour and clinical trials have shown low-level effectiveness, with no adverse reactions: though allergy to shellfish would be a contraindication.

Herbal and vitamin supplements

Herbal supplements are numerous. Examples include echinacea, ginger, ginkgo biloba, garlic, devil's claw, nettles, celery seeds, feverfew, ginseng and willow. Emu oil is sold as a topical application. The claimed modes of action differ: some are said to stimulate the immune system, so are marketed as remedies for illnesses such as influenza. Feverfew is claimed to have specific effects on blood vessels and inflammation and is marketed for migraine as well as arthritis. Aspirin is a salicylate, regarded as a manufactured medication but which was originally derived from willow.

Vitamin supplementation of a balanced diet containing fresh fruit and vegetables should be unnecessary. However, many ill patients are not taking such a diet, so in selected cases, vitamin supplements may be necessary. This is best decided in conjunction with a health professional.

Q I keep reading that I should eat a healthy balanced diet, but I don't really know what that is. I know about too much animal fat, red meat and cream; I eat fresh fruit almost every day and we do not over-cook vegetables. What else should I eat or avoid? Someone told me that I have arthritis because I am allergic to something in my diet: How do I find out?

A You are doing the right things, so far as we know. There have been claims of various forms of arthritis being caused by food. However, documented cases are few and far between. Milk allergy causing stomach upsets, chest problems or headaches in infants and also adults, is of course well known. However, there have been only a handful of convincing cases where the diagnosis of, say, rheumatoid arthritis has been confirmed and then a dietary change has been followed by a permanent remission of the inflammation. The process of proving food allergy takes the patience of a saint. For at least a whole month you would have to consume a diet containing nothing but bland foods such as carrots, lamb, rice and spring water from glass bottles. Presuming that the arthritis has settled down (which of course may be due to a natural variation in symptoms) you would then have to introduce one candidate food at a time for a few days at a time. This process takes ages. Then there is the question of measurement of symptoms and the placebo effect. This process is so laborious that there have been very few scientific studies.

> ### Q What about probiotics?
>
> **A** Probiotics are currently all the rage. There may well be a place for these in condition such as coeliac disease, after an attack of tropical diarrhoea, or during prolonged antibiotic therapy, but no one (yet) has claimed efficacy for arthritis. Then there is the question of claimed reactions to colouring additives and food preservatives. There are to date no convincing and repeatable instances of arthritis being caused by such constituents – but there is always the possibility of a first!

It seems most likely that many of these herbal remedies or dietary supplements do have a modicum of therapeutic benefit, in at least a proportion of patients. However, it should be remembered that the more powerful the potential benefit, then the more powerful the possible toxicity. Interference with prescription medication has been known to occur with some preparations, so any patient considering taking such supplements would do well to read thoroughly all the accompanying literature, as they may well not be able to seek advice on this particular compound from a pharmacist or doctor.

At best, these dietary modifications and supplements appear to offer a symptomatic, 'NSAID' effect. There has been no convincing and repeated evidence that any of them offer a 'disease-modifying' therapeutic benefit although such cases may exist. Perhaps they do not come to the notice of doctors specializing in the field, who would be very willing to consider and write up convincing cases of cure of RA with such a supplement or dietary modification.

Complementary medical professionals

Homeopathic, Ayurvedic, traditional Chinese medical practitioners and others practise according to well-established principles using systems of examination and ethical codes of practice. Well-qualified complementary practitioners will not hesitate to recommend conventional medical advice if the situation demands it. However, trials of homeopathic treatment have shown conflicting results. For conditions such as fibromyalgia, mild osteoarthritis (OA) or mild, non-progressive inflammatory arthritis it is reasonable that a patient wishing to avoid conventional medication, as discussed below, tries the benefits of such treatments. However, a patient with an active and potentially serious form of rheumatic disease would be well advised firstly to inform their doctor at the outset and, secondly, not to continue the complementary route if they deteriorate progressively. That is not to say that conventional medical treatment is always effective: it is not, and it does have very definite potential risks, as will be described.

The medical treatment of arthritis: what can a patient expect?

When a patient with rheumatic or arthritic symptoms consults a doctor, she (or he) can reasonably expect to be listened to and to be examined. Blood tests and other investigations may follow. A working diagnosis, or at least an appraisal of the problem and some suggestions as to the possible diagnoses, should result. A referral to a rheumatologist is not by any means

myth
'Treatment' means having to take medicines.

fact
The word 'treatment' covers a number of things, which may include taking medicines. But health problems such as arthritis require a dialogue and understanding between doctor and patient as to what can be achieved, with or without medication.

always required. As has been indicated, rheumatic problems are very common. Mostly, they do not require specialist referral. However, for severe cases of common conditions such as osteoarthritis and for virtually all inflammatory arthritis or systemic rheumatic disease, a rheumatological referral is likely to be advisable. It may not be necessary for follow-up to be prolonged: a single consultation may be all that is required for, say, gout or non-progressive ankylosing spondylitis (AS).

Ice, heat and TENS machines

Pain is debilitating and depressing. Physical means of coping with pain range from ice and heat to the use of TENS (Transcutaneous Electrical Nerve Stimulation) machines. An illustration of the consequences of long-term local heat for pain relief can be seen in figure 10.2. Extremes of temperature do seem empirically to help: presumably by altering the appreciation of pain through the nervous system. Anyone who has been working outside in icy weather and banged a freezing finger end with a hammer will remember how agonizing the pain can be! Any football fan will have seen the physio rush onto the field with a freezing spray to get some player back on their feet. One can buy special wheat bags to stick in the freezer for cold or in the microwave for warmth. A few minutes experimentation will demonstrate which if any is the better for aching joints. Trials have shown that for gout ice packs are better at relieving the intense pain of an acute gouty toe than heat: the gouty joint is perhaps hot enough! Whereas for some people with osteoarthritis ice is preferable, and for others it is

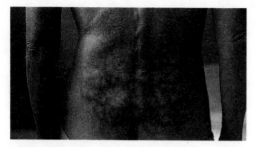

◖ Figure 10.2 Chronic back pain heat marks.

warmth. Physiotherapists use infrared light therapy, which warms tissues, rather like a heat lamp. It is uncertain how TENS exerts its pain relieving effect but it is likely that it stimulates the body's own pain suppressants, endorphins. Perhaps it has an effect on the brain, like acupuncture. The electrodes are placed on the surface of the skin and a tiny current passes through them for several hours, gradually relieving pain in the area beneath.

Acupuncture

The ancient Chinese technique of acupuncture was regarded with a mixture of wonder and even derision until quite recently. However, it has spread from the private medical sector to the National Health Service in the UK, where it is now quite widely practised in pain clinics and physiotherapy departments. Whether it becomes as readily accepted in the UK as it is in China remains to be seen. It is moderately but definitely effective in osteoarthritis of the knee, so presumably it will also relieve pain in other joints as well. Its appropriate place in the treatment of other forms of arthritis remains to be found. There is no evidence that it changes the nature or progress of the underlying arthritis.

Analgesics

Analgesics or painkillers, such as paracetamol, are the most widely used and still the mainstay of treatment of OA. Dosages of six to eight tablets per day may be required, although it is preferable to keep the dose lower than that. Most preparations of plain paracetamol for adults are of 500 mgm. However, stronger preparations are available from pharmacies so always check the dosage, whether it be a tablet, powder or liquid. The total dosage should not be more than 4 g per 24 hours for an adult, less for a child or frail person. Combinations of paracetamol with codeine are also commonly used, so check that you are not taking, for example, a flu remedy which contains paracetemol in conjuction with your plain paracetamol. The combination with dextropropoxyphene (Co-proxamol) is being phased out because of the number of inadvertent or deliberate overdoses. It is not a good idea to use aspirin as a daily analgesic because of its irritant effect on the stomach, producing bleeding and also bruising or asthma in the unwary. Low-dose aspirin, as used to prevent strokes, will not have a detectable analgesic effect.

Other analgesic preparations such as dihydro-codeine, nefopam, or tramadol are used for arthritis in selected instances. Pethidine or morphine are also used, although rarely required for arthritis on a regular basis.

All analgesics tend to produce side-effects such as drowsiness and nausea. Constipation is common with codeine.

NSAIDs remain in common use. There is a wide range, including ibuprofen, diclofenac, naproxen and piroxicam. They also continue to provide problems due to their side-effects on the stomach and also the kidney. It was for a time hoped that the Coxib drugs, such as Vioxx, would retain the effectiveness of NSAIDs, while reducing the impact on the stomach through their selective inhibition of the inflammatory mediator Cox-2. Unfortunately it has become apparent that, while the gastric problems have certainly been fewer, their potential for causing heart problems has led to the withdrawal of two and doubts about this group of drugs as a whole. Patients may, however, be reassured that the added risk of a heart attack or stroke due to taking one of the NSAID group of drugs, including the Coxib drugs, is very small indeed. It is, for example, far outweighed by smoking, raised cholesterol, previous heart attacks or uncontrolled blood pressure.

Q **I cannot take diclofenac for the arthritis in my thumbs because of stomach pains. Codeine makes me constipated. What else could I take for my arthritis?**

A This is a common problem. Sometimes the effects on the stomach are offset by taking a drug such as cimetidine or omeprazole, but taking one drug to counter the side-effects of another is not an ideal approach. Other painkillers such as tramadol are possibilities. It is also worth considering using one of the NSAID gels, such as diclofenac gel or ibuprofen gel, rubbed in regularly to the affected joints. While not very powerful, this may take the edge off the pain. Capsaicin gel has also been shown to work. Unlike the NSAID gels, it works by a sort of counter-irritation.

Try to become an expert on your own medication – after all, you are the one who is taking it! It is also worth remembering the following:

✧ mistakes can happen: pharmacists, doctors and nurses are only human, so always read the leaflet accompanying any new medication that is prescribed to make sure that it is what you think it is going to be

✧ read the label on every new bottle of medication you receive to make sure there has been no error in type or dosage

✧ take note of the dosage

✧ never put tablets into other bottles then change the labels

✧ be wary of borrowing someone else's medication, even if it seems identical to yours.

Disease-modifying and immunosuppressive drugs

The DMARD drugs and immunosuppressives, including methotrexate, cyclophosphamide, aza-thioprine, cyclosporine and anti-TNF (tumour necrosis factor) drugs have been considered earlier. Here we shall consider steroids.

Corticosteroids are still in widespread use, both orally and by injection, in a wide range of doses. The 'folk memory' of their problems is considerable, and some patients are put off any thought of taking them. On the other hand, familiarity breeds contempt, so it is worthwhile discussing them here in more detail. Predni-solone will be used as the main topic, since the principles apply to any of the other similar compounds.

Oral prednisolone comes in tablets of:

✧ 1.0 mgm – white
✧ 2.5 mgm – white

- 2.5 mgm – brown coated to reduce stomach upset – although the downside to this coating is that they may not be as well absorbed
- 5.0 mgm – white, not soluble in water
- 5.0 mgm – red coated, see above
- 5.0 mgm – white, soluble in water.

You can see why it is very important that you understand your medication and read the labels! If you cannot do so, it would be wise to find someone else to.

Steroid side-effects

These are many and varied. The commonly known ones are the tendency to make you put on weight, by stimulating appetite (some people start eating like horses) and by causing fluid retention. Also well known is the effect of precipitating or worsening diabetes and of increasing blood pressure. Less well known is the effect of producing wakefulness during the first week or two of treatment. This can be quite unsettling, although it will improve with time. Some people actually feel quite odd and de-personalized or agitated. Another effect of longer term treatment, especially in older people, is the steroid bruising shown in figure 10.3.

Osteoporosis is mentioned in Chapter 5 in relation to RA. It is relevant to any condition in which steroids are prescribed. In particular, people with polymyalgia rheumatica (PMR) (Chapter 7, page 157) are prone to develop osteoporosis, because they tend to be older and may already have thin bones. Spontaneous osteoporosis is discussed in Chapter 9 (page 169).

Q **I have a condition called Polymyalgia. My doctor says that I should be treated with steroid drugs or else I might go blind. But my aunt was treated with steroids and nearly went blind because the steroids apparently caused cataracts. I am confused and a bit frightened: what should I do?**

A This is a very understandable predicament. Firstly, the risk of going blind if you don't take steroids is low: see Chapter 7. However, it is true that there is very little likelihood of it settling down without steroids. Secondly, steroids can indeed cause cataracts. However, this is not a high risk because the doses used are quite low. Also, cataracts can be treated quite successfully nowadays.

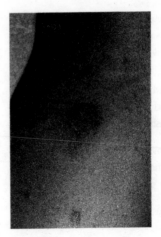

❚ Figure 10.3 Steroid bruising.

Steroid injections

These are used for soft tissue problems such as tennis elbow or shoulder pain. They are also useful as part of the plan for treating acute flare-ups of inflammation such as in RA or lupus. The injections may be given into muscle intravenously or into the joint or soft tissue. The intramuscular and intravenous preparations have been discussed in Chapters 5 and 7, but it is worth reiterating a few points here.

There is no absolute definition, but a moderate dose might be anything over 30 mgm of prednisolone, which can usually be given orally (i.e. by mouth). A large dose, anything over 100 mgm, is usually given intramuscularly. A 'pulse' or 'bolus' dose is 500 mgm or above, usually given intravenously. The intramuscular and intravenous preparations are usually of methylprednisolone. The doses given into a joint are from 10 to 15 mgm, when given into tiny joints such as the finger, up to 50 mgm into a knee. The preparations mostly in use are hydrocortisone, prednisolone, triamcinolone or methylprednisolone.

The general points to consider with joint injections are:

✧ the dose and indication (i.e. the reason for the injection)
✧ the frequency of injection
✧ the potential risks.

The reason for an injection into a joint, bursa or tendon is really up to the treating physician or surgeon in discussion with the patient. It is rather surprising how often there is benefit, for example in osteoarthritis, when at the time of examination there does not seems to be much inflammation present. Yet sometimes, when there is clearly inflammation, there seems to be lamentably little benefit. On the whole, however, steroid injections do provide good benefit for a limited period of time. This benefit may last from a week to several weeks. In fact, especially when the arthritis is varying, that benefit may appear permanent. So it is difficult to specify how frequently injections into the same joint should be given. A figure of a maximum of three per year is often quoted, but that is based on experience and pragmatism rather than evidence.

The greatest potential risk from steroid injections into joints is infection. If a patient has any current skin infection, certainly if it is near the part to be injected, the injection should usually be deferred. Sometimes there is a redness at the site or even a temporary apparent flare for a few hours or a day following an injection, but any pronounced redness and pain at rest should be assessed by a doctor as soon as possible, in case infection has occurred. This is extremely rare, but

Q **Are joint injections painful?**

A The anticipation is usually the worst aspect, especially if you have not had one before. An injection into a joint should not be painful, although even in expert hands, it occasionally is. The skin can be anaesthetized with an anaesthetic spray, then local anaesthetic (provided you are not allergic) is slowly injected to numb the capsule of the joint, which is the most tender part. If a large needle has to be used in order to draw off fluid, the likelihood of pain is greater. On the other hand, the relief of pain as the fluid is extracted will be considerable! If no fluid needs to be drawn off, a thin needle can be used; when using one of these, there is often no need for anaesthetic and there is very little risk of bleeding.

can happen and should always be borne in mind. There are well-established protocols when administering steroid injections for ensuring this risk is very low.

A less well-known risk of steroid injections is wasting of soft tissue or de-pigmentation of the skin at the site of the injection, leaving a thinned-out area of skin (see plate 12). This is more likely to happen if long acting steroids such as methylprednisolone are used, for example, for tennis elbow, or if the injection is repeated several times at the same site.

Damage to joints can occur from very high doses of steroids given by mouth, by injection or intravenously. This is called avascular necrosis but it can also occur spontaneously during illnesses such as lupus.

Steroids are rightly regarded with some trepidation by patients but they can offer powerful benefits. If steroids had no side-effects, we would probably need no other drug with which to suppress unwanted inflammation.

CHAPTER

11

Investigations and laboratory tests

A diagnosis may result from the symptoms given by the patient and the subsequent physical examination, but some form of investigation often follows. In general, investigations are carried out in order to:

✧ throw more light on symptoms and the results of physical examination
✧ detect any hidden disorder
✧ screen for problems that might be relevant in the future
✧ rule out specific conditions
✧ monitor the effects of treatment.

The investigations that are most frequently relevant to arthritis are summarized in the table on next page. Some laboratories may perform different but equivalent tests. There are of course many other tests that are less often carried out in patients with arthritis.

Blood test	Includes	Purpose
Full (total) blood count (FBC)	Haemoglobin (Hb)	Detection of anaemia
	White blood cells (WBC) Total and differential count of types of white cell; platelets	Detection of types of infection/inflammation and state of bone marrow
Erythrocyte sedimentation rate (ESR)	A single test	Measures inflammation
C-reactive protein (CRP)	A single test	Measures inflammation
Urea and electrolytes (U & E)	Levels of creatinine, urea, sodium, potassium	Assesses kidney function
Liver function tests (LFT)	Liver enzymes Alkaline phosphatase Albumen, bilirubin	Assesses liver function
Autoantibody tests	Rheumatoid Factor (RF)	Assessment of arthritis and autoimmune disease
	Anti-nuclear antibody (ANA)	Detection of autoimmune disease
	Anti-ENA (antibody to extractable nuclear antigens)	Assesses type of autoimmune disease
	Anti-DNA	Diagnosis and progress of systemic lupus erythematosus (SLE)
	Anti-neutrophil cytoplasmic antibody (ANCA)	Diagnosis and type of vasculitis

Many of the tests are fairly self-evident, but here are further explanations of some that may cause confusion.

ESR versus CRP

The ESR (erythrocyte sedimentation rate) is a non-specific test. It is done on whole blood, including the red cells, the white cells and the plasma, so it is a composite of lots of changes in the blood. For example, it goes up if there is anaemia because of changes in the red cells (red corpuscles) or during pregnancy. The healthy level is up to about 15 or 20 mm per hr (millimetres per hour). There is some variation with age. It cannot distinguish between infection and inflammation, as it goes up with both and it also goes up if there is an abnormality of the serum proteins. It responds rather slowly (over several days or more) to changes in the intensity of inflammation and drops slowly after an infection is cured.

The CRP (c-reactive protein), on the other hand, is a very specific protein. It is measured in plasma or serum, so is independent of the haemoglobin and cells in the blood. It rises extremely rapidly and does not last long in the blood, so drops again quickly once the infection or inflammation settles down.

Rheumatoid Factor (RF)

This is an autoantibody: it is an antibody made in the body, like the antibodies that are made in response to infection. It is a sort of an antibody to an antibody. It is positive in cases of rheumatoid arthritis (RA) that are likely to remain active and might be damaging, but is only moderately useful in making a prediction as to how severe the arthritis is likely to be. It is not a test for arthritis. Some patients can have quite severe arthritis with a negative test. It can occur in normal healthy people, especially those who have a relative with RA, so it should not be over-interpreted.

Anti-nuclear antibody (ANA – formerly called ANF)

This autoantibody, that reacts with nuclear material from cells, is found in low concentrations in many healthy people, especially as they get a bit older, so the conditions under which the test is done have to be quite robust in order to be sure that it is not a coincidental finding. Even then, it does not necessarily imply severe disease. It will detect autoimmune diseases, but does not indicate clearly the type.

The ENA (antibody to extractable nuclear antigens)

This test is carried out to help decide what sort of autoimmune condition the patient has. For example, there are different types of ENA in Sjögren's syndrome, scleroderma and inflammatory muscle disease.

Anti-DNA

This is an antibody to DNA itself, which is very weird. There are various ways of carrying out the test, some of which are very specific for systemic lupus erythematosus (SLE) and also vary with disease activity, especially of kidney disease in SLE.

Anti-neutrophil cytoplasmic antibody (ANCA)

This is an autoantibody to certain cell contents and is useful both to diagnose and to follow the activity of systemic vasculitis.

Imaging

Imaging means taking pictures. This usually means static pictures, especially where arthritis is concerned. So they look at anatomy as distinct from physiology, biochemistry or immunology, as do blood tests.

X-rays

The soft tissues are not seen well on X-rays and it is the soft tissues that hurt, so these are useful for seeing any damage that has accumulated, rather than interpreting symptoms. Often there are abnormalities that give no symptoms at all, or are irrelevant to the present problem. X-rays of the spine, for example, are a very poor way of assessing back pain symptoms.

Ultrasound scanning

Just as this technique is used for examining the liver or the uterus, the soft tissues around joints can be examined, to get a better view of swelling or soft tissue tears.

CT scanning (computerized tomography)

This still involves X-rays, but enables a more precise view of tissues.

MRI scanning (magnetic resonance imaging)

MRI does not use X-rays, so the risks are less. It is a very complex and expensive bit of equipment but has improved diagnosis a great deal.

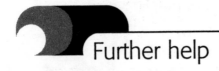

Further help

Useful addresses

Arthritis Care
18–20 Stephenson Way
London
NW1 2HD
Tel: 020 7380 6500
Fax: 020 7380 6505
http://www.arthritiscare.org.uk
(Provides advice on social benefits
and welfare assistance,
information booklets, courses for
patients)
Email: info@arthritiscare.org.uk

Arthritis Research Campaign
Copeman House
St Mary's Court
St Mary's Gate
Chesterfield

Derbyshire
S41 7TD
Tel: 0870 850 5000
Fax: 01246 558007
Email: info@arc.org.uk
http://www.arc.org.uk
(Medical research charity which
funds research into all types of
arthritis, also provides information
for the public and doctors and
other health professionals)

Back Care
16 Elmtree Road
Teddington
TW11 8ST
Tel: 020 8977 5474
Fax: 020 8943 5318
Helpline: 0845 130 2704
http://www.backcare.org.uk

(National Back Pain Association)
(Represents both patients and
health professionals dealing with
back pain. Provides information and
support and promotes self-help)

British Sjögrens Syndrome Association
PO Box 10867
Birmingham
B16 0ZW
Tel: 0121 455 6532
http://www.bssa.uk.net

http://www.arthritis.ca/types
(Canada)

Complementary medicines
www.quackwatch.org/index.html

Diets
http://www.oilofpisces.com/
rheumatoidarthritis.html
(See also *Diet and Arthritis* by Dr
G. Darlington, published by
Vermillion)
http://www.marketresearch.com/
map/prod/1099196.html
http://www.mindbranch.com

Fibromyalgia Association UK
PO Box 206
Stourbridge
West Midlands
DY9 8YL
Fax: 0870 752 5718
http://www.fibromyalgia-
associationuk.org

STIFF UK (Support Through Information for Fibromyalgia Family and Friends)
PO Box 1484
Newcastle-under-Lyme
Staffordshire
ST5 7NZ
Tel: 01782 562366
(as a call-back service
11a.m.–4p.m.)
http://www.stiffuk.org

General information
http://patients.uptodate.com – a
comprehensive guide with a lot of
detail to all sorts of illnesses,
including rheumatic disorders

Gout
UK Gout Society
http://www.ukgoutsociety.org

LUPUS UK
St James House
Eastern Road
Romford
Essex
RM1 3NH
Tel: 01708 731251
Fax: 01708 731252
http://www.lupusuk.com
headoffice@lupusuk.org.uk
This is a useful website from an
American Lupus support group:
http://www.mtio.com/lupus/
lal_1.htm

National Ankylosing Spondylitis Society
Parkshot House
5 Kew Road
Richmond
Surrey
TW9 2PR
Tel: 020 8334 7026
Email: nass@nass.co.uk
http://www.nass.co.uk

National Rheumatoid Arthritis Society (NRAS)
Unit B4 Westacott Business Centre
Westacott Way
Littlewick Green
Maidenhead
Berkshire
SL6 3RT
Helpline: 0845 458 3969
General number: 01628 823524
Email: enquiries@rheumatoid.org.uk
http://www.rheumatoid.org.uk

Psoriasis Association
7 Milton Street
Northampton
Northants
NN2 7JG
Tel: 0845 676 0076

Fax: 01604 792894
http://www.psoriasis-association.org.uk
(Aims to support those who have psoriasis, raise awareness about psoriasis and fund research into the causes of and treatments for psoriasis)

Raynaud's & Scleroderma Association
112 Crewe Road
Alsager
Cheshire
ST7 2JA
Tel: 01270 872776
Freephone: 0800 917 2494
(for UK enquiries only)
Fax: 01270 883556
Email: info@raynauds.org.uk

Soft tissue rheumatic disorders Work-related upper limb disorders
http://www.hse.gov.uk/pubns/
http://www.hcd2.bupa.co.uk/fact_sheets/html

Vasculitis
http://www.vasculitis.med.jhu.edu

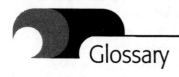

Glossary

μ = micro

acute inflammation	this may refer to a recent and short lived reaction to injury, burns or infections and is characterized by pain, tenderness, redness and swelling
aggrecan	a chemical component of cartilage
alopecia	loss of hair – usually just patchy thinning in lupus
anaemia of chronic disease	anaemia due to inflammation or infection, not due to iron deficiency
analgesic medication	painkilling tablets, injections or patches (the noun is 'analgesia')
ANCA (anti-neutrophil cytoplasmic antibody)	autoantibody found in patients with systemic vasculitis
annulus fibrosus	strong rim around each intervertebral disc in the spine
anserine bursitis	inflammation of the anserine bursa, which is just below the inner aspect of the knee
antibody	an immunoglobulin protein that sticks to an antigen, such as a bacterium

antigen	a protein that sticks to antibody forming an immune complex
anti-nuclear antibody (ANA)	an autoantibody positive in 95–8% of patients with lupus
arthralgia	painful joints
atherosclerosis	the furring up of arteries that causes heart attacks, strokes or, as used here, pain in the leg muscles when walking. This is called claudication (named after the Latin for 'to limp').
autoimmunity and **autoimmune disorder**	when the body's immune system is over-active in certain specific ways, creating abnormally large amounts of antibody proteins, such as Rheumatoid Factor or anti-nuclear antibody, and also specific reactions against the body's own tissues, such as thyroid
avascular necrosis	the impairment of blood supply to a bone, usually within a joint, causing it to collapse. Can occur spontaneously or can be caused by very high doses of corticosteroids.
balanitis	inflammation or infection of the end of the penis
bisphosphonate	drug for treating osteoporosis.
Bursa (plural = bursae)	cushioning sac or double-sided membrane over a bony prominence
bursitis	bursitis means inflammation of a bursa, which is a thin double-sided membrane a bit like an uninflated balloon that allows one tissue to glide easily over another. Typically, bursae are situated around bony prominences such as the elbow, knee, shoulder or hip.
calcaneal spur (heel spur)	common bony outgrowth at the heel at the insertion of the *plantar fascia*
calcium pyrophosphate deposition disease (CPPD)	inflammatory arthritis due to calcium crystals; can resemble gout (hence 'pseudo gout'); occurs in osteoarthritis
cervical spondylosis	osteoarthritis of the neck
cheiragra	gout in the hand
chondroitin	a chemical component of cartilage

chronic inflammation	may look similar to acute inflammation, but long-lasting and with different microscopic features
cimetidine	drug to reduce stomach acid secretion
claudication	limping, due to poor blood supply
collagen	the main component of connective tissue throughout the body, including cartilage and tendon
complement	part of the body's initial defence against infection; part of the immune system
coronary thrombosis	heart attack
corticosteroid	see *steroids*
crepitus	crunchy noise and sensation within joints or tendons
CRP	C-reactive protein: part of the infection defence system; rises rapidly with infection and many types of inflammation
cruralgia	the equivalent of sciatica, but with pain and numbness at the front of the thigh and knees
CT	computerized tomography
cyclophosphamide	drug used in cancer therapy, but also suppresses immunological inflammation
cytotoxic drug	a drug that kills cells. This usually means malignant (cancerous) cells, but in inflammatory conditions as in this book, it means the suppression or killing of cells of the immune system
discoid lupus	type of lupus rash
diuretic	drug used to relieve fluid retention
DMARDs	disease-modifying anti-rheumatic drugs
Dupuytren's	fibrous contracture in the hand
ENA	extractable nuclear antigen: test for sub-types of diseases related to lupus
endocrine glands	these are glands such as the thyroid or adrenal, that secrete hormones into the blood stream

endorphins	body chemicals that help to suppress pain
enthesis	the junction or insertion of a ligament or tendon into bone
enthesitis	term used to describe the tissue where a ligament, a tendon or a joint capsule merges with or is inserted into a bone
ESR	erythrocyte sedimentation rate: this measures inflammation, infection or abnormalities in serum proteins
exocrine glands	these are glands that secrete substances, such as the salivary glands that make saliva
familial juvenile hyperuricaemic nephropathy	rare kidney condition in children, that results also in gout
fascia lata	strong flat ligament down the side of the thigh
FBC	full blood count
Felty's syndrome	unusual complication of rheumatoid arthritis, with blood abnormalities
foramen	the little tunnel or space through which a nerve passes as it emerges from the spine out into the adjacent tissue of nerve bundle e.g. the sciatic nerve
Forestier's syndrome	advanced variant of spinal osteoarthritis
full blood count	haemoglobin (for anaemia), total white blood cell count and differential white cell count (predominantly neutrophils and lymphocytes), platelet count
glucosamine	a chemical component of cartilage
gonagra	gout in the knee
granulomatous	type of chronic inflammation
hallux rigidus	stiffening of the great toe
haematological	blood related
haemolytic anaemia	a type of anaemia involving destruction of red cells
Heberden's nodes	osteoarthritic bony swelling of joints at the end of the finger
heparin	anti-coagulant drug, given intravenously

hepatomegaly	enlargement of the liver
hyperuricaemia	raised uric acid (urate) level in the blood
immunoglobulin	antibody protein involved in defence against infection but also in chronic immunological conditions
inflammation	the reaction to injury, burns, infections, characterized by pain, tenderness, redness and swelling. In the context of this book, it refers to apparently spontaneous inflammation arising in joints or associated tissues. *Acute inflammation* means recent and short-lived; *chronic inflammation* means long-lasting.
ischaemia	shortage of blood supply
keratoderma blenorrhagica	a rash, resembling psoriasis, which appears on the soles of the feet in Reiter's Syndrome
ketosis	an acid condition of the body which gives a sour smell on the breath
Lesch-Nyhan syndrome	rare inherited disease, with mental deficiency and gout
ligament	strong tissue that joins bones together and limits the movement of a joint; consists mostly of collagen
livedo reticularis	a reddish-purple rash usually found over the extremities
lordosis	normal inward curve of the spine
lupus	short for Systemic Lupus Erythematosus (see page 210)
lupus profundus	type of lupus rash
lymphadenopathy	enlarged lymph nodes (lymph glands)
lymphopoietic system	lymph nodes, spleen, liver
monitoring	this refers to the regular taking of blood tests or other investigations, to pick up drug side-effects
MRI	magnetic resonance imaging
MSM methylsulfonylmethane	a sulphur compound that is sold as a patent medicine for many diseases
myocardial infarction	heart attack

myopathy	a muscle disorder. This can include inherited muscle disease or inflammation (myositis). It can also be caused by medication, such as prolonged treatment with high doses of steroids.
myositis	inflammation of muscle
nephritis	inflammation of the kidney
neutrophils	white cell subtype
Nifedipine	drug used for blood pressure control
nodules	little firm swellings found in rheumatoid arthritis
nucleus pulposum	centre of intervertebral disc
oedema	the accumulation of fluid in soft tissue
oesophagus	gullet
olecranon	tip of elbow
Osgood-Schlatter's disease	a form of osteo-chondritis at the lower end of the patellar tendon at the knee; occurs in adolescent growth
osteo-chondritis	mild inflammatory condition of growing joints and bones
osteophyte	bony outgrowth in osteoarthritis
osteoporosis	reduced density of bone
pauci- or oligo-articular arthritis	arthritis affecting a few joints – usually five or fewer
pathological	related to disease or, sometimes, just to severe symptoms
pericardial effusion	fluid in the sac around the heart
pericarditis	inflammation of the sac around the heart
periosteum	the thin membrane which covers a bone and provides cells which aid healing of fractures
phagocytic	process of white cells engulfing debris or bacteria
phospholipids	membrane fatty protein
phosphoribo-sylpyrophosphate synthetase superactivity (PRPs) syndrome	Rare metabolic disorder, causing gout
photosensitivity	undue sensitivity to sunlight
pilocarpine	drug sometimes used to reduce saliva secretion

placebo	tablet containing no effective medication
plantar fascitis	pain and inflammation of the plantar fascia, the strong ligamentous structure that stretches along the sole of the foot
platelets	tiny corpuscles involved in clotting
pleura	lining around lungs
pleural effusions	fluid in pleura
pleurisy	inflammation of pleura
pneumonitis	inflammation of lungs
podagra	gout in the foot
polyangiitis	inflammation of blood vessels
polymorphonuclear leucocyte	subtype of white blood cell – a first-line defence against infection
pre-eclampsia	disorder that can occur in pregnancy, with raised blood pressure and protein in the urine. It can be dangerous for both the baby and the mother and needs urgent assessment and treatment.
pre-patellar bursitis	inflammation of the bursa at the front of the knee
prostacycline	biological produce affecting blood vessel function; used to treat spasm of blood vessels
proteoglycans	a chemical component of cartilage that attracts water and swells
proton pump inhibitors	reduce acid secretion in stomach
pulmonary fibrosis	fibrosis of lungs
pulmonary hypertension	raised pressure within the lung circulation
purpura	purplish rash due to little patches of bleeding into skin
pyrophosphate	a chemical substance that occurs normally throughout the body. However, especially with advancing age, it may accumulate in joint cartilage as crystals. These can sometimes cause inflammation. This may be acute or similar to gout – hence the term 'pseudo-gout'. Or a rather more grumbling inflammation may develop. Also

	known as pyrophosphate deposition disease (see *CPPD*).
Raynaud's phenomenon	reversible spasm of blood vessels, normally in the fingers
reflux	stomach acid coming up the gullet
Reiter's syndrome	a combination of arthritis, bowel or genitourinary infection and eye inflammation – one of the spondylarthropathy group
reticulo-endothelial system	this is made up of the lymph nodes, liver, spleen and bone marrow
RF	Rheumatoid Factor
rotator cuff muscles	supraspinatus, infraspinatus and subscapularis: muscles which control shoulder movements
sacroiliitis	inflammation of the sacroiliac joints, which join the pelvis to the spine
sciatica	pain and/or numbness and/or pins and needles radiating from the buttock down the side of the leg to the toes. It is usually not a continuous radiation of pain: there is often a 'gap' of normal sensation down the side of the thigh and knee, with the emphasis being at the side of the calf. This is because the commonest nerve root to be involved is the fifth lumbar nerve root, which supplies sensation to the outer calf.
septic arthritis	infection of a joint by a bacterium. Reactive or infection associated arthritis is arthritis developing because of an infection, but where the organism is not actually found in the joint
Sjögren's syndrome	a rheumatic condition characterised by inadequate saliva and tears along with rheumatic and other symptoms
sphincter	type of valve
spinal stenosis	narrowing of the space for the nerves within the lumbar spine
splenomegaly	enlargement of the spleen

spondylosis	osteoarthritis of the spine – especially used in cervical spondylosis (of the neck) or lumbar spondylosis (of the lower back)
sternum	breastbone
steroids	a group of hormone chemicals, occurring naturally in the body but also made into drugs for the treatment of several types of condition. The word should not be confused with the type of steroid used and abused by some sportsmen and bodybuilders. In this book, the word is used as short-hand for corticosteroids, which reduce inflammation.
Stickler syndrome	a rare inherited condition of collagen, which results in various degrees of eye problem and a type of premature osteoarthritis
syndrome	any collection of signs and symptoms
synovium, synovial membrane	lining of a joint
systemic	this term is used quite loosely. It may refer to a medical condition involving more than one system of the body (e.g. skin and heart), as in Systemic Lupus Erythematosus or Systemic Vasculitis. It is also used to indicate when a person feels generally ill, such as in the term 'systemically unwell'. Infections such as rubella are described as systemic because the patient is generally ill, whereas a boil in the skin, which is also an infection, is by definition quite localised, so may not give rise to feeling generally unwell.
systemic lupus erythematosus (lupus, SLE)	a condition which can give rise to a wide range of symptoms, including arthritis, fevers, skin rashes and kidney problems
tendon	strong tissue that runs from the end of a muscle to a bone; made mostly of collagen
thrombosis	clot
TNF (tumour necrosis factor)	protein involved in inflammation

tophus (plural tophi)	collection of uric acid crystals which present as swellings
uric acid/urate	the end product of purine breakdown in the human
uricase	an enzyme that breaks down uric acid to form a more soluble compound, called allantoin. Uricase is present in most animal species but humans have lost it through evolution, so they can get gout!
uricosuric	drug causing excretion of uric acid
urticaria	an itchy rash
vasculitis	inflammatory disease of blood vessels
vasodilators	drugs that open up blood vessels
warfarin	anticoagulant drug: anti-clot
WBC	white blood cell count
white cell count	white blood cell count

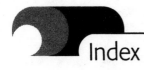

Index

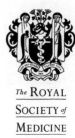

The ROYAL
SOCIETY of
MEDICINE

The Royal Society of Medicine (RSM) is an independent medical charity with a primary aim to provide continuing professional development for qualified medical and health-related professionals. The public benefits from health care professionals who have received high quality and relevant education from the RSM.

The Society celebrated its bicentenary in 2005. Each year it arranges and holds over 400 meetings for health care professionals across a wide range of medical subjects. In order to aid education and further training the Society also has the largest postgraduate medical library in Europe – based in central London together with online access to specialist databases. RSM Press, the Society's publishing arm, publishes books and journals principally aimed at the medical profession.

A number of conferences and events are held each year for the public as well as members of the Society. These include the successful 'Medicine and Me' series, designed to bring together patients, their carers and the medical profession. In addition, the RSM's Open and History of Medicine Sections arrange meetings on a regular basis which can be attended by the public.

In addition to the lectures and training provided by the RSM, members of the Society also have access to club facilities including accommodation and a restaurant. The conference and meeting facilities of the RSM were refurbished for their bicentenary and are available to the public for hire for meetings and seminars. In addition, Chandos House, a beautifully restored Georgian townhouse, designed by Robert Adam, is also now available to hire for training, receptions and weddings (as it has a civil wedding licence).

To find out more about the Royal Society of Medicine and the work it undertakes please visit www.rsm.ac.uk or call 020 7290 2991. For more information about RSM Press, please visit www.rsmpress.co.uk.